# Health Needs Assessment

*For Churchill Livingstone:*

*Commissioning editor*: Ellen Green
*Project development editor*: Mairi McCubbin
*Project manager*: Valerie Burgess
*Project controller*: Derek Robertson
*Copy editor*: Paul Singleton
*Indexer*: Laurence Errington
*Design direction*: Judith Wright
*Sales promotion executive*: Hilary Brown

# Health Needs Assessment
## Theory and Practice

**Jane Robinson** FRCN MA PhD MIPM RGN ONC RHV HVT
Department of Nursing and Midwifery Studies,
Faculty of Medicine and Health Sciences, University of Nottingham, UK

**Ruth Elkan** BA (Hons)
Department of Nursing and Midwifery Studies,
Faculty of Medicine and Health Sciences, University of Nottingham, UK

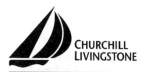
CHURCHILL
LIVINGSTONE

NEW YORK EDINBURGH LONDON MADRID MELBOURNE SAN FRANCISCO TOKYO 1996

CHURCHILL LIVINGSTONE
Medical Division of Pearson Professional Limited

Distributed in the United States of America by Churchill
Livingstone, 650 Avenue of the Americas, New York, N.Y.
10011, and by associated companies, branches and
representatives throughout the world.

First published 1996

ISBN 0 443 05233 6

**British Library Cataloguing in Publication Data**
A catalogue record for this book is available from the
British Library.

**Library of Congress Cataloging in Publication Data**
A catalog record for this book is available from the Library
of Congress.

The
publisher's
policy is to use
**paper manufactured
from sustainable forests**

Produced through Longman Malaysia, PP

# Contents

# Preface

*Health Needs Assessment* began life in response to a demand for teaching materials in an area which the Project 2000 reforms of nurse education placed firmly on the educational agenda. When the idea was first mooted at the beginning of 1992, it seemed a relatively straightforward matter to consider producing a book on epidemiology and public health for nurses which would address some of the educational needs raised by *Project 2000: a New Preparation for Practice* (United Kingdom Central Council of Nursing, Midwifery and Health Visiting, UKCC, 1986). The Project 2000 Report had examined the question of whether health needs in 20 years time were likely to differ from those of the late 1980s and had concluded that because, in future, more health care would be delivered in the community, nursing would be less hospital-based and nurse education should reflect that change. The Project Group recommended therefore that pre-registration nurse education and training should be re-oriented towards the community, with less emphasis on hospital care, and that the education focus should shift to the wider context of health production and promotion. In nurse education of the future, the treatment of disease should be seen as one part of a broad context of pre-disposing factors, prevention, incidence, diagnosis, possible cure and rehabilitation.

While the focus of the book was under discussion we realised that policy developments in the National Health Service (NHS) and elsewhere had overtaken us. The division of the NHS into purchaser and provider functions following the implementation of the 1990 NHS and Community Care Act meant that health needs assessment had become much more complex. For a variety of reasons, which we shall explore in *Health Needs Assessment*, the process had become dependent on a variety of other influences and perspectives – lay and theoretical, professional and policy-oriented. Furthermore, there was no general agreement on how to choose any one 'best way' from the numerous ways of viewing and *doing* health needs assessment which were being advanced from different quarters. This situation left us with a considerable dilemma as to what to include in our proposed book. We recognised the impossibility of writing a straightforward 'cookbook' for nurses on how to 'do' health needs assessment without acknowledging the current debates and unresolved difficulties surrounding the subject. The alternative was to try to encompass some of these diverse issues.

It was this alternative which we chose to follow. We wanted a book which would assist nurses (who in practice already carry out a great deal of health needs assessment at grass roots in the community) to grasp the complex context of current issues surrounding the process of needs assessment so that they could contribute to the debates and develop their practice appropriately. Hence we took the decision to address both practical and theoretical perspectives. The result is a book in which practical approaches to health needs assessment are described but which also considers the ethical, economic, epidemiological and sociological literature on the subject, together with an analysis of some of the policy initiatives which have given rise to Government pleas for a mixture of expertise *and* pragmatism in the face of so many unresearched problems in the field of health care. An inevitable consequence of our decision is that *Health Needs Assessment* is not a *textbook* on how to carry out the activities involved, because what emerges from the many different views on how health needs assessment can be carried out is the variety of approaches which are possible. Instead, we have given examples of how others have carried out health needs assessment for different purposes and have given sources which provide a wide range of examples of particular forms of assessment. In this way we believe that we have given nurses and other health care professionals access to a variety of tools from which they can make informed choices when they themselves are involved in the process of health needs assessment.

As we have said, *Health Needs Assessment* began life as a pragmatic response to the needs of the nursing professions for material in this area. We now believe that this *alternative* book, concerned as it is with the diverse theoretical perspectives on which needs assessment activity is based, together with a description of some of the difficulties involved in their application to practice, will be of interest to a much wider audience. We should point out that this is a rapidly evolving field. During the later stages of the preparation of *Health Needs Assessment* a quite substantial modification to the government's approach to equity and health became apparent (see Ch. 4), and two papers were published which demonstrated that other nursing and social policy analysts were following similar lines of inquiry to ourselves (Billings & Cowley 1995, Lightfoot, 1995).

## The need for a knowledge base for health needs assessment

Perhaps unsurprisingly, the new purchaser/provider culture in the NHS has revealed that in many instances the *knowledge and skills* on which to base rational decision-making for commissioning are restricted to a narrow band of experts in their respective fields, or are simply not available at all. Hence the Government has given substantial amounts of policy guidance on how to proceed. For example, on health needs assessment as a basi for service planning; in the *Health of the Nation* strategy for the setting of priorities and targets; and in setting up a central research and development function within the NHS in order to address many of the current unknowns within health care (for example, Department of Health 1991a,b, 1992, 1993a, Welsh Office 1995).

Close inspection of official documents reveals however that these policy initiatives are not always based on a uniform set of ideas. *Health Needs Assessment* sets out to describe and to analyse the theoretical positions from which these contemporary policies are derived. 'Analysis' is used here in the sense which indicates that judgement is suspended while a review of the background to a policy issue, including its origins and affiliations, is explored. This may be a relatively new perspective for readers of texts written for health care practitioners (especially nurses) which tend, in general, to offer 'facts' rather than critical reviews and/or reflection on policy issues. We defend this shift in perspective on the grounds that health needs assessment is an activity based on *theories* which often conflict, rather than complement each other. We would have found it impossible to write a book on health needs assessment without acknowledging the current difficulties surrounding the subject.

We hope that health care practitioners will be reassured rather than confused when they read of the different views which can be drawn

# Acknowledgements

In writing this book we have received support from a number of people. We would like to thank Margaret Reid, Department of Public Health, University of Glasgow, for her constructive comments on the book, and Pippa Gough, Professional Officer, UKCC. We would also like to thank Elizabeth Hart, Department of Nursing and Midwifery Studies, University of Nottingham and Meg Bond, Department of Continuing Education, University of Warwick for their helpful comments on an early draft of Chapters 2–7. Many thanks are also due to Jane Wolstenholme, Trent Institute for Health Services Research and to Walter Elkan for their helpful comments on Chapter 7.

We would also like to thank in particular the following current and former undergraduates in the Department of Nursing and Midwifery Studies, University of Nottingham, for allowing us to use extracts from their Bachelor of Nursing Neighbourhood Studies: Jill Connell, Sharon File, Alison Hibberd, Rebekah Howe, Shamin Khalik, Claire Miskella, Kathryn Parbhoo, Joanne Preston, Jean Procter, Rachel Savage, Emma Watson, Frances Wiseman.

Finally, thanks to Robbie Robinson for his patience and encouragement.

# Abbreviations

| | |
|---|---|
| BMA | British Medical Association |
| CHD | Coronary Heart Disease |
| CMO | Chief Medical Officer |
| DHA | District Health Authority |
| DPH | Director of Public Health |
| FHSA | Family Health Service Authority |
| GHS | General Household Survey |
| HVA | Health Visitors' Association |
| NAHAT | National Association of Health Authorities and Trusts |
| NHSE | National Health Service Executive |
| NHSME | National Health Service Management Executive |
| NDU | Nursing Development Unit |
| OPCS | Office of Population Censuses and Surveys |
| PREP | Post-Registration Education and Practice |
| QALY | Quality Adjusted Life Year |
| RCN | Royal College of Nursing |
| RSHG | Radical Statistics Health Group |
| SMR | Standardized Mortality Ratio |
| SNMAC | Standing Nursing and Midwifery Advisory Committee |
| UKCC | United Kingdom Central Council for Nursing, Midwifery and Health Visiting |
| WHO | World Health Organization |

# Who assesses health needs?

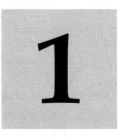

## INTRODUCTION

We begin by introducing *who* carries out health needs assessment at a local level. We consider the contributions of professional health care workers, voluntary and community groups, and social and economic scientists. We conclude Chapter 1 by setting out the structure of the book.

## WHO ASSESSES HEALTH NEEDS?

The systematic assessment of need prior to any form of health care intervention, whether with individuals or groups, lies at the heart of all research-based professional education and practice and, since 1989, population health needs assessment has been strongly endorsed by Government initiatives (see Ch. 4). Under the 1990 NHS and Community Care Act District Health Authorities (DHAs) and local authorities respectively are required to assess health and social needs as a means of obtaining accurate and appropriate information on which to base policy (Hawtin et al 1994). The division of the NHS into 'purchaser' and 'provider' functions, together with a sharpening of policy focus on the cost-effectiveness of the services purchased and provided, has resulted in a greater awareness among health care practitioners of the requirement not only to assess need as a means of defining the precise objectives of their service, but also to identify the most efficient means by which those objectives might be achieved. We begin by giving some examples of the contributions to local health needs assessment made by health care practitioners, community groups and social scientists.

## Directors of public health

Public health physicians are the professional group who, historically, have had the overall, formal responsibility of assessing population health needs within the British health care system. The principle tool of public health physicians is epidemiology (see Ch. 6) and although epidemiology is not the sole preserve of the medical profession it has emerged historically as a medical speciality. By tradition, epidemiology in the British context has developed since the middle of the last century as part of the public health function under the auspices of government Chief Medical Officers of Health (CMO). Every year the CMO produces an Annual Report, currently entitled *On the State of the Public Health*. The Report for 1993 is the 136th in the series which began in 1858 (Department of Health 1994). Like its predecessors, the Report covers a broad range of health matters of immediate national concern or interest, including vital statistics, health policy, health care, communicable diseases and environmental health. CMOs have always worked closely with their colleagues (currently known as Directors of Public Health, DsPH) who head local public health departments. Previously known as Medical Officers of Health, DsPH were based prior to the 1973 NHS Act with local government departments and, after 1974, with Regional and District Health Authorities (Public Health in England 1988). (The environmental health function has remained with local government departments, the responsibility of County and City Councils.)

In 1988, the Committee of Inquiry into the Future Development of the Public Health Function in England stated that the public health responsibilities of DHAs are so important that they should be the responsibility of a single, named, leader known as the Director of Public Health ([DPH], Public Health in England 1988). The Committee defined the central tasks of the DPH and his/her colleagues as follows (Public Health in England 1988, pp. 69–70):

1. to provide epidemiological advice to the District General Manager (DGM) and the DHA and the setting of priorities, planning of services and evaluation of outcomes;

2.  to develop and evaluate policy on prevention, health promotion and health education involving all those working in this field. To undertake surveillance of communicable disease;
3.  to co-ordinate control of communicable disease;
4.  generally, to act as chief medical advisor to the authority;
5.  to prepare an annual report on the health of the population (or to quote the former Medical Officer of Health [MoH] duty 'To inform himself as far as practicable respecting all matters affecting or likely to affect the public health in the [district] and be prepared to advise the [health authority] on any such matter');
6.  to act as spokesperson for the DHA on appropriate public health matters;
7.  to provide public health medical advice to and link with the local authorities, Family Practitioner Committees (FPCs) and other sectors in public health activities.

Like their CMO counterpart at national level, many DsPH produce their own annual reports on health matters of contemporary concern in their local DHA. Hence, by tradition, public health and epidemiology has come to be seen as a medical speciality. In Chapter 10 we shall look at practical ways in which one DPH carried out part of her DHA responsibilities for health needs assessment through the publication of annual reports.

## Non-medical epidemiologists

Medical doctors who choose public health as a career study for the degree of Master in Public Health (MPH) in university departments of public health medicine and epidemiology. Academic departments of public health medicine in universities, together with government agencies such as the Public Health Laboratory Service are also important sources of epidemiological research. However, epidemiology is carried out increasingly by non-medical personnel, including statisticians, microbiologists, medical geographers and, in the study of disease patterns over time, historians. Increasing numbers of non-medical personnel (including nurses) now undertake the MPH, and the principles of epidemiology and public health are included in many non-medical health care practitioners' second level courses. Nurses working in purchasing authorities, such as District Health Authorities and Family Health Service Authorities, are involved increasingly in the epidemiological assessment of need prior to the setting of contracts.

## Health visitors and community nurses

In recent years, community nursing staff have become increasingly proficient in the development of community and case load profiles which include 'bottom up' approaches to the epidemiological assessment of need. Curricula for courses for health visiting, district, school and, increasingly, practice nursing now include the concepts of health needs assessment for the particular populations within the nurses' remit. The introduction of PREP by the UKCC will ensure that, in future, all community nursing courses include a common foundation programme which will result in a consolidation of epidemiological and public health principles for nurses who choose to work in the community (UKCC 1994). The implementation of Project 2000 for the first-level education and training of nurses in the United Kingdom, with its focus on the factors which influence states of health and disease, now ensures that these principles are introduced from the very beginning of nurse education.

The formalization of group and population-based health needs assessment by nurses working in community settings can be traced from 1965, when a new syllabus of training for health visitors was introduced (Council for the Education and Training of Health Visitors 1965). Subsequent description of the function of the health visitor included the 'Recognition and identification of need and mobilization of appropriate resources' (Council for the Education and Training of Health Visitors 1967). These initiatives were followed by an investigation into the principles of health visiting which described four principles for practice: 'The search for health needs; the stimulation of the awareness of health needs; the influence on policies affecting health; and the facilitation of health enhancing activities' (Council for the Education and Training of Health Visitors 1977, p. 9). These principles were developed into practice as health visitors began what has now become routine in many health authorities, to carry out health needs assessments in geographical areas, or with general practice populations. As district nurse, and then school nurse education, moved into higher education the principles of health needs assessment were gradually adopted and modified for these particular branches of community nursing. The Health Visitors' Association

(HVA) now publishes guides to various aspects of health profiling (Twinn et al 1990, Blackburn 1992a, b, Health Visitors' Association School Nurse Sub-Committee 1992). In Chapter 11 we shall give some examples of local health needs assessments by health visitors.

## Nursing and health care students

Today, in the 1990s, *all* nurses following the Project 2000 model of nurse education, whether at diploma or degree level, begin their nursing careers with a grounding in social and community health (UKCC 1986). Many Project 2000 pre-registration courses require students to carry out some form of health needs assessment, either as a neighbourhood study or community profile. The tradition which nurses have developed of assessing health needs at the level of the individual and their families through the use of the nursing process is therefore being extended to include an analysis of the wider social context for health. The purpose of this extended learning lies in the belief that an understanding of the wider context of health and disease can enhance the quality of nursing and health care. Nurses are not alone, for these educational shifts are also reflected in the education of medical students and the therapy professions. Student health care practitioners working in both hospital and community settings are now being provided with the tools to appreciate that many of the characteristics of the patients they meet, and the diseases with which they present, form part of a complex pattern of individual and community health. Health care can thus be more sensitively assessed and appropriately delivered. In Chapter 11 we shall give some examples of local health needs assessments carried out by undergraduate student nurses.

## All members of the nursing and midwifery professions

More recently, key proposals from the report *Making it Happen* (Standing Nursing and Midwifery Advisory Committee 1995) state that nurses, midwives and health visitors should be viewed as key workers in strategies for improving the health of the population and not solely as professionals delivering specific health services to individuals. The base line of these strategies is the prior assessment of need against which to measure the success of interventions. The Standing Nursing and Midwifery Advisory Committee (SNMAC) believes that all nurses, midwives and health visitors have a major role to play in improving public health because:

- the scale of their contacts with the population provides unparalleled opportunities for promoting health;
- they meet a wide cross-section of society;
- they work in a variety of settings: homes, schools, workplaces, hospitals, the community and other environments;
- they have privileged access to information about personal health, which can inform the assessment of health needs;
- they can communicate health information to a very large number of people;
- they are valued by society;
- they are part of a diverse range of professional and voluntary networks.

  (National Association of Health Authorities and Trusts 1995, p. 1)

While recognising the traditional contribution of nurses working outside institutional boundaries to community health, the Standing Nursing and Midwifery Advisory Committee (SNMAC) report also points to ways in which other areas of nursing are developing their contributions to improved public health. These contributions include:

- nurses' involvement in clinical audit activity and the development of profiles against which to assess effectiveness;
- school nurses, midwives' and practice nurses' wide range of health promotion work;
- nurses in mental health and learning disabilities work in enabling clients to participate in strategic and operational decisions in the services to which they relate;
- occupational health nurses' work in screening and the promotion of positive health, especially in men;
- secondary care nurses' involvement in early detection of illness and treatment, rehabilitation and palliative care.

### Examples of good practice
The SNMAC 1995 report gives examples of the good practice which it envisages could become much more widespread among nursing. The examples include:

- a nurse working from a DHA Public Health Department involved in health needs assessment and managing the strategic purchasing

programme for elderly people and people with physical
disabilities;

- a public health nurse in an NHS Trust focusing on improvements
to local determinants of health in a disadvantaged city area;
- a health visitor working with homeless people;
- a staff nurse in intensive care who developed and evaluated an
accidental injury awareness programme for local school children;
- a communicable diseases control nurse working in a large city
with a commercial port, contributing to the monitoring,
surveillance, prevention and control of infection throughout the
DHA and planning and investigating major incidents involving
outbreaks of infection, accidental release of chemicals, and
radiation leakages;
- a Community infection-control nurse managing a team of nurses
who work across the DHA/local authority structures for
environmental control, contact-tracing, and vaccination and
immunization for mobile groups.

## Nurses in purchasing authorities

Many of the ideas for the expanded role of nurses put forward by
the SNMAC report are also reflected in The Department of Health
and the National Health Service Management Executive (NHS
Management Executive) suggestions that although much of nursing's
contribution to patient care is in provider units (including community
units) it is essential not to overlook the contribution which the
nursing profession can make in purchasing organizations (NHS
Management Executive 1993a, pp. 15–16, NHS Management Executive
1993b, p. 45, NHS Executive 1994, Department of Health 1995a). The
NHS Management Executive argues that if the targets to improve the
nation's health set out in the *Health of the Nation* (Department of
Health 1992, NHS Management Executive 1993c,d) are to be achieved
(see Ch. 4), and if there is to be more patient choice and improvements in the quality of services, then the nursing professions must
have an effective involvement in commissioning and purchasing. In
its document entitled *A Vision for the Future*, the NHS Management
Executive (1993a) suggests that there are a number of areas in which
appropriately skilled nurses, midwives and health visitors can make
a valuable contribution in purchasing organizations:

First, their knowledge of patterns of illness and disease and treatment regimes enable them to work alongside Directors of Public Health and other colleagues to assess the health needs of populations, and the impact of health interventions.

Second, the communication skills which many nurses, midwives and health visitors acquire during their professional education can equip them to participate in consultation with groups and individuals about their health needs and to feed back to the community information about purchasing decisions made on their behalf.

Third, in negotiating contract specifications the experience which nurses and midwives have in provider settings enables them to contribute to drawing up both the qualitative and quantitative elements of specifications, and can also help their managerial and finance colleagues interpret an array of sometimes conflicting clinical data.

Finally, in evaluating and monitoring services delivered against contract, nurses midwives and health visitors can play a key part in ensuring the maintenance and improvement of measurable standards of care, and the achievement of health care targets and outcomes. (NHS Management Executive 1993a, pp. 15–16, paras 3.32–3.34)

## NEEDS ASSESSMENT IN COMMUNITY HEALTH

The assessment and collation of information relating to local health needs is the bottom rung of a ladder for the development of wider community health profiles, for example at DHA level, all of which serve to influence local and national policy. As the Government documents referred to above point out, the importance of practitioners' active participation in the community for the collection and generation of local knowledge cannot be overestimated. Sharing in the provision of local health services forms part of the warp and the weft of community life and nurses and other community health and social workers gain tremendous insights into the strengths, needs and problems of the individuals and groups who make up the local population. Health care practitioners working in the community therefore have a considerable advantage over researchers like Frankenberg (1969) whose publication *Communities in Britain: Social Life in Town and Country* was on the reading list of many community nursing courses during the 1970s. In the Introduction (p. 16), Frankenberg writes:

When I went to Glynceiriog I was always conscious of my anthropological colleagues' anecdotes of how they sat in the centre of African villages while life went on around them and encompassed them. They could not avoid becoming part of the social processes they wished to observe. In my early days in the village I would often climb a hill and look sadly down upon the rows of houses of the housing estate and wonder what went on inside them. When I became involved in the affairs of the football club and other activities which concerned the village as a whole, I too was able to observe social process but never as intensely as my Africanist colleagues .... By and large (students of areas of this kind) can only deduce social process .... by questioning people in their homes or elsewhere. For there are no activities which concern the estate as a whole.

Health workers, in contrast to Frankenberg's account, frequently *are* participants in local community activities. Through their contribution to the delivery of local health care and by the application of epidemiological, psychological and social science principles and knowledge, they act both as community participants *and* as local researchers. Through their close involvement with groups and individuals in the community a comprehensive picture of the health strengths and needs of the populations for which they have responsibility can be constructed. These assessments, when taken together with all other forms of health needs assessment carried out by other agencies in the community, can then form the basis for review and recommendations for changes in policy.

## The contribution of voluntary and community groups

Health needs assessment is not the sole prerogative of professional groups. Voluntary and community groups frequently present evidence on the existence of unmet needs, or lack of resources, as essential parts of their campaigns for or against a particular development (such as the building of a new hospital, or bed closures) (Hawtin et al 1994). The contribution of voluntary and community groups to needs assessment is an example of the need to adopt a practical approach to issues when faced with the reality of assessing need at a local level. At the end of the day, politicians, health care professionals and consumer groups charged with the responsibility for defining and providing health care services, have to *act* by making choices which involve taking difficult, often political, decisions. Each group may have justifiably different concerns. Politicians may give priority to an economic perspective which places cost-effectiveness, if not cost reduction, at the centre of policy. Consumer groups may be concerned primarily with the rights of individuals to have equitable access to health care (see Ch. 5). Health care professionals may try to reconcile both perspectives within the overriding ethic of a Duty of Care to the groups and individuals for whom they provide a service (see Ch. 7). What frequently emerges is a compromise which, at best, will maximize the opportunities for health gain from available resources. Pragmatics is concerned with adopting a practical approach to issues, and it appears that the pragmatics of health needs assessment invariably involves a measure of negotiation and compromise between potentially competing interests. Voluntary and community groups are more likely therefore to adopt community action forms of health needs assessment where the empowering of local people, or groups with special needs, is seen as a crucially important step in ensuring that their views as service users are taken into account when political or professional decisions are made.

At the end of their book *Community Profiling: Auditing Social Needs*, Hawtin et al (1994) include an annotated bibliography which includes useful examples of community profiles produced by: Citizens Advice Bureaux; church groups; community action groups; health authorities and community health councils; independent consultants; local authorities; profiles for political purposes; self-study profiles; and profiles by universities, polytechnics and colleges.

## The contribution of social scientists

A large part of *Health Needs Assessment* is concerned with making explicit the interrelationship between different underlying theoretical perspectives and current health needs assessment practice and policies. Chapters 2 to 7 are concerned in different ways with the application of a variety of theories (epidemiological, economic, ethical and sociological) to the practical concerns of assessing and delivering cost-effective health care. By acting in a pragmatic way, key actors involved in the process of assessing health needs (whether professionals, politicians, or citizens) sometimes lose sight of the theoretical under-pinnings for their practical acts. It is a key concern of this book that in reminding readers that these connections *really* exist, they should also be aware of the very real *tensions* and *problems* which arise when one attempts to apply theories *uncritically* to any area of practice. The dangers are particularly acute when assessing health needs for, as the remainder of the book will show, the practice of health needs assessment is dependent on a wide variety of theories, many of which do not mesh easily with one another when it comes to their *practical* application.

In Chapter 2 we shall discuss Bradshaw's important contribution to the clarification of the concept of 'need' (Bradshaw 1972a,b, 1994) and the vastly different views held by economists and theorists such as Doyal & Gough (1992) on the subject of whether or not the concept of 'objective need' actually exists. Fitzpatrick (1995) has made explicit some of the social sciences' distinctive contributions, including the importance of emphasizing the sufferer's own perspective regarding his or her illness. In discussing the contribution of the social sciences to a specific area of health needs assessment, namely the assessment of chronic illness Fitzpatrick also highlights some of the difficulties associated with applying social science knowledge to everyday practice and the potential pitfalls which await any practitioner who attempts uncritically, or too enthusiastically, to apply a tool or construct developed in an experimental situation, or in theory, to an everyday practice situation.

Fitzpatrick's warning of the problems involved in the assessment of chronic disease (see Ch. 3), demonstrates an important but frequently overlooked contribution of the social sciences to health needs assessment. This is the ability to disentangle and look critically at the complex components of an issue, and to encourage people to reflect on the dangers of assuming an oversimplistic view of social reality. This is one of the central messages that we would hope *Health Needs Assessment* will convey. It is not that having to handle so many different perspectives leads to a paralysis of action, but rather that it helps to inject a note of realism into the process and an understanding of the need for a degree of compromise in the face of so many competing claims.

All health needs assessment concerns three central elements: health problems (need), resources, and outcomes (health gain). Throughout the remainder of this book it will be seen that none of these elements is unproblematic. Even the authors cited in this chapter, who are pragmatic realists in their approach to health needs assessment, recommend that the task should be undertaken in different ways and give greater emphasis to one aspect rather than another.

## THE STRUCTURE OF *HEALTH NEEDS ASSESSMENT*

Despite the pragmatic approach, the ways in which needs and health gain (or outcomes) are viewed still depends therefore very much on implicit underlying theoretical perspectives. These are the elements which we shall begin to introduce throughout the remainder of the book. Chapter 2 introduces different definitions and key perspectives on health needs assessment. In Chapter 3 we shall consider the issues involved in the definition and measurement of health needs. Chapter 4, on the approach of central government, examines how government policy in the Health of the Nation strategy has attempted to reconcile the often conflicting perspectives put forward by the epidemiological and economic health disciplines, and presents some of the criticisms which have been levelled at the policy as a result. Chapter 4 also looks at central government guidance to District Health Authorities in assessing health needs. Chapter 5, on inequalities in health, explores the relationship between health and the socio-economic circumstances of people's lives and considers the different theories which have been developed in order to *explain* health inequalities. It will be seen that, when applied, these theories lead to very different policy implications; creating further dilemmas for policy makers. Chapters 6 and 7 explore further the very different approaches to health needs assessment advanced respectively within the disciplines of epidemiology and economics. Chapter 8 considers screening as a very specific approach to health needs assessment and shows that despite the major influence of epidemiological perspectives in developing screening programmes, economic concepts of *cost* are also of vital importance when deciding whether or not a screening programme should be introduced. Chapters 9 to 11 return to the theme of practical, local, health needs assessment. Chapter 9 explores the central elements which appear to some extent in all local health needs assessments – health problems, resources and outcomes – and how four sets of authors have used these elements in their own approaches to the subject. Chapters 10 and 11 are based on examples of work carried out in Nottingham. Chapter 10 examines the discharge of the statutory function of the Director of Public Health (DPH) in presenting an assessment of the health needs of the people of Nottingham prior to the District Health Authority's (DHA) purchase of health care services. Chapter 11, after reference to a rare empirical study on consumers' views on health needs assessment, reports on local health profiling by health visitors at the Strelley Nursing Development Unit (NDU) and on work carried out by undergraduate nurses in the first two years of their Bachelor of Nursing (Hons) degree. It is argued that if similar activity is being carried on by nurses and health visitors around the country, then contemporary government policies for local health needs assessment are already being met by many members of the nursing professions. Chapter 12 concludes with a reflection on the implications for nurses of the theoretical and practical aspects of health needs assessment.

The practical examples given throughout *Health Needs Assessment* do not *solve* the theoretical dilemmas but help to demonstrate how issues are addressed when health care practitioners are faced with competing conceptual perspectives on health problems, and a requirement to *act* in the real world of need and demand.

# Key perspectives on the assessment of health needs

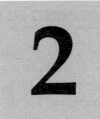

## INTRODUCTION

Health needs assessment is underpinned by a range of different theoretical and ethical perspectives. It is doubtful whether some of these very different approaches can ever be reconciled, but Black (1994) has suggested that some kind of balance must be found between competing perspectives and objectives: 'We need a balance between what *should* be done in terms of need; what *can* be done at a practical clinical level; and what can be *afforded*; for this we need a combined economic, clinical and ethical appraisal'. Black thus summarizes the basic elements of health needs assessment. He suggests that meeting health needs is a moral or ethical question, a question of what we as a society value, and what goals or outcomes we desire to bring about. He points out that what we *can* do in practice is limited by the knowledge and skills we currently possess (some illnesses can be cured or at least treated successfully, others cannot). And finally he stresses the fact, unpalatable to many, that it is not possible to do all that we can and should do because there are limits to the resources at our disposal.

This chapter introduces some of the basic concepts and theories underlying differing approaches to health needs assessment. These are all explored further in subsequent chapters. We begin by looking at definitions of health needs assessment.

## DEFINING HEALTH NEEDS ASSESSMENT

One way of defining health needs assessment is as a process of measuring ill-health in a population. Under this definition health needs are viewed as health losses, and health needs assessment involves the construction of a health profile (or rather an illness profile) which, in turn, relies on measures of the incidence, prevalence and degree of severity of various health problems in the population. The greater the amount of ill-health the greater is need (Pickin & St Leger 1994, Mooney 1994).

There are two main difficulties with this definition. The first is that not all health needs are health losses. People who are not ill have a need to remain well; they have a need to be protected as far as is possible from ill-health. The second shortcoming of this definition is that it says nothing about what is to be done once health problems have been identified. It implies (but does no more than imply) that once health problems have been identified they can be solved. However, not all health problems can be solved. Some curative interventions extend life, or restore normal functioning, others do not. Some 'caring' interventions enhance the quality of life but others do not. Some interventions designed to ensure that people remain well are successful, others less so. Thus some interventions are more effective or beneficial than others.

A second, more sophisticated definition of health needs is the 'capacity to benefit from health care'. In this definition health needs are not health problems, they are the capacity to benefit from health-related interventions. The amount of need is not dependent on the size of the health problem (the incidence and prevalence of ill-health). The amount of need is dependent on the ability to benefit from health-related interventions. The greater is the ability to benefit, the greater is need. This second definition is much in vogue at the present time. As we shall see in Chapter 4, it is the definition currently favoured by the government and the National Health Service Executive.

One advantage of this second definition over the first is that it recognizes that not all health problems can be successfully treated or cured. There is the recognition that some conditions respond better than others to health-care interventions (Mooney 1994). A second advantage of this second definition is that it forces us to look at what outcome we desire to achieve. If need is 'the capacity to benefit', then we have to say what it means to benefit. There are many possible benefits of health care. Benefits can include both those which extend life, adding 'years to life', and those which enhance the quality of life, adding 'life to years' (Department of Health 1992); moreover, they can include not only physical but also psychological and social benefits. Thus, under this second definition it is not enough to identify a health problem as amenable to some kind of intervention or treatment. We must also spell out what sort of outcome or benefit the intervention is intended to bring about. This second definition thus acknowledges that health needs assessment involves value-judgements about what outcomes or benefits we desire to pursue. Crucially, it raises the question of who decides what is a beneficial outcome, since there is often a disparity between, for example, the judgements of professionals and lay people about whether a particular intervention is beneficial (Jenkins 1990). This is discussed further below and in subsequent chapters of the book.

One drawback of this second definition is its blunt but inescapable logical conclusion that if people do not have the ability to benefit in any way whatsoever from the treatments and services currently on offer then they are not in need. Even where people do have some capacity to benefit, their capacity to benefit may be inversely related to the severity of their health problem. For example, if 'capacity to benefit' is defined narrowly as the capacity to achieve a longer life, then a person with moderately severe heart disease may have a greater capacity to benefit from coronary by-pass surgery than someone with very severe heart disease whose life may not be greatly extended by such surgery. It is the effectiveness of the treatment rather than the severity of the health problem which determines whether one person is in greater need than another. The first definition has some advantages here, in that clearly there *are* people with health problems for whom current treatments are ineffective, but about whom it nevertheless makes sense to say that they are in need. For example, it makes sense to say that people with incurable illnesses such as motor neurone disease, or AIDS, are in need. Culyer (1977) deals with this drawback of the second definition by suggesting that what people with health problems unamenable to any kind of health intervention need is research. Those who currently have no, or very little, capacity to benefit from health-care interventions are still in need, but they are in need of successful research rather than ineffective treatments.

A second drawback of the definition of need as the 'capacity to benefit' is that in practice, benefits are often defined in a narrow way by clinicians, researchers and policy makers, who may concentrate only on interventions which can be shown to be effective in extending life, or in restoring normal functioning, rather than on interventions which aim to provide high quality palliative care or to increase social and psychological support to patients and their carers. People with motor neurone disease or AIDS may have only a limited capacity to benefit from curative interventions, but they certainly have the ability to benefit from caring interventions.

A third drawback of the 'ability to benefit' definition relates to the question of who is to decide what is a beneficial outcome. Pickin & St Leger (1994) point out that a definition of need as the 'ability to benefit' often leads to an approach to health needs assessment which starts by looking at the services currently available and only then looks at how many people and what sorts of people might benefit from them. Pickin and St Leger urge that we focus initially on people and not on services if services are to be appropriate to people's needs. They stress that we need to know what sorts of outcomes people value, what sorts of benefits they hope to receive. We cannot rely on what those providing services judge to be others' capacity to benefit (Pickin & St Leger 1994).

A third perspective on health needs assessment is supplied by health economists. Health economists are not happy with either of the above two definitions. They prefer the second to the first because it acknowledges that we cannot meet all health needs (Mooney 1994). However, they point out that the capacity to benefit from health services is always going to be far greater than the resources at our disposal to implement every possible beneficial intervention. It is economists who stress that we must choose between beneficial outcomes, we must choose who is to receive a beneficial service and who is not (Williams 1993a): 'No society can afford to offer all its members all the health care that might possibly do them some good. Each society has therefore to establish priorities, that is, it has to decide who will get what and, by implication, who will go without'.

Thus, for economists, health needs assessment cannot be divorced from the question of rationing. If health care resources are to be allocated on the basis of 'need' or on the basis of an 'ability to benefit' from health care, this in turn means determining priorities between competing claims on limited resources. Not all these competing claims on health care resources can be met and therefore health needs assessment must inevitably result in some form of rationing.

## HEALTH AND HEALTH CARE

What is often referred to as 'health needs assessment' is, strictly speaking, 'health-care needs assessment'. Health, or the absence of ill-health, is not dependent solely on health care services. These are only one determinant of health. Health also depends on such things as appropriate nutrition and housing, a safe physical environment, economic security, and a social and psychological environment which fosters emotional security and a sense of self worth and belonging. Health is affected by many interventions outside the health care services. It is affected by individuals themselves (for example, through diet, or behaviour such as smoking). It is also affected by road safety policies, clean air and other public health measures, and by occupational health and safety regulations (Mooney 1992). It is affected by policies to reduce poverty and unemployment. It is affected, too, by the kinds of social relationships in which people's lives are embedded. Health is thus determined by much more than health care services (Pickin & St Leger 1994). A full health needs assessment would require that all health-related policies and measures, and not simply health-care services, be taken into account. As we shall see in Chapter 4, many statutory organizations, such as District Health Authorities (DHAs) confine their activities largely to an assessment of health-care needs. Although DHAs recognize the wide range of influences on health, it is their statutory role to meet health-care needs rather to meet the full range of health needs. By contrast, health needs assessment exercises undertaken by, for example, community groups or by nurses, often address a much wider range of influences on health.

## THEORETICAL APPROACHES TO 'NEED' AND THEIR IMPLICATIONS FOR PRACTICE

In the following section we examine various theoretical approaches to the concept of need, and their implications for the practice of assessing health needs.

## Bradshaw's typology of need

An important early attempt to define 'need' was undertaken by Bradshaw, a sociologist. Although Bradshaw's concern was not specifically with *health* needs, his work is nevertheless of relevance in clarifying differing definitions of need. Bradshaw (1972a,b) outlined four separate types of need:

### 1. Normative need

This is what the expert or professional or administrator defines as need in particular situations. A standard is laid down, and if people fall short of the standard they are identified as in need. Examples are the British Medical Association's (BMA) nutritional standard which is used as a normative measure of the adequacy of a diet. Normative definitions of need are not absolute; they may change as a result of changes in knowledge and changing values. There may be different, even conflicting, standards laid down by different experts. Normative definitions of need have faced the charge of elitism or paternalism.

### 2. Felt need

Felt need is equated with want. When assessing the need for a service, people are asked whether they feel they need it. In a democracy, Bradshaw suggests, it might be thought that felt need was important, but in reality felt need is often not taken into account. 'Felt need', Bradshaw suggests, is an inadequate measure of 'real need' because it is limited by the individual's perceptions of his/her needs. People might not know that there is a service available – they will not feel a need for something which they do not know exists. Moreover, people may be reluctant to admit to a loss of independence – they may not acknowledge to themselves or others that they are in need. On the other hand, there are those who may ask for help without actually needing it.

### 3. Expressed need

This is felt need turned into action. Expressed need is what economists call the demand for a service. People do not demand services unless they feel they need them, but it is common for felt need not to be expressed by demand. Expressed need is commonly used as a measure of need by health service planners. For example, waiting lists are often taken as a measure of expressed need or demand. However,

Bradshaw points out that waiting lists are generally accepted as a poor definition of 'real need', especially for pre-symptomatic conditions where people neither feel, nor therefore express, a need.

## 4. Comparative need

Comparative need is found by studying the characteristics of those already in receipt of a service. If one person with similar characteristics to another is not receiving the same service, then that person is in need. This definition can be used to assess the needs not only of individuals but also of groups of people. For example, a great deal of research has been carried out to identify those characteristics, such as low income, unemployment, and lone parenthood which are associated with poor health (see Chs 3 and 5, 10 and 11). Comparative need at a population level is the difference between the services provided in one area and those provided in another, weighted to take account of the factors known to increase the risk of poor health. 'Comparative need' is thus about equity (Bradshaw 1994). It is about equal provision for equal need and unequal provision for unequal need. This is discussed further in Chapter 5 where we look at the concepts of 'horizontal' and 'vertical' equity.

One difficulty with the concept of 'comparative need' (and with the principles of 'horizontal' and 'vertical' equity) is to determine which are the significant characteristics to be taken into account in assessing comparative need. A second difficulty is that the services which are provided (the 'supply') may still not correspond with need. If population $A$ is in need in comparison with population $B$, this does not necessarily mean that population $B$ is thereby not in need. The supply of services to population $B$ may not be at an adequate level.

Bradshaw's work is useful at both a theoretical and a practical level. At the theoretical level it is useful in drawing attention to the fact that different definitions of 'need' correspond with different groups in society. 'Normative need' reflects the value-judgements of professionals and experts, while 'felt need' embodies the values of individuals.

Bradshaw's work is also of great practical value. In order to illustrate how his typology can be used by those engaged in the practical task of assessing needs, Bradshaw discusses a hypothetical example of a Local Authority wishing to assess the housing needs of its elderly population (Bradshaw 1972a).

### Case study: Bradshaw's approach to the assessment of the housing needs of the elderly

In Bradshaw's hypothetical example, a research worker is commissioned by a Local Authority to assess the housing needs of the elderly population. The research worker gathers information about the needs of the elderly under each of the four separate definitions of need given below.

**Normative need.** In Bradshaw's hypothetical example, the Local Authority has laid down certain norms. It has decided that old people living in homes lacking any of the basic amenities, and those living in overcrowded accommodation are in need. Bradshaw suggests that an estimate of the number of people living in this situation could be obtained by means of a sample survey. (We would add that the Census is also a very useful source of this type of information.)

**Felt need.** An estimate of the extent of felt need could be obtained by means of the same sample survey by asking people whether they were satisfied with their current housing, and whether or not they would like to move. Bradshaw stresses that it is important to take account of the factors which affect people's attitudes. He points out that elderly people's responses to questions about their housing needs will be affected by their knowledge of alternative housing provision, as well as their worries about the upheaval involved.

**Expressed need.** In this situation, the measure of expressed need is the Local Authority's waiting list. However, Bradshaw stresses that waiting lists can be a poor measure of need. They may overestimate expressed need if they are inflated by people who have already found alternative accommodation but whose application has not been withdrawn. Conversely, they may underestimate expressed need if certain groups are excluded from the waiting list – for example, those who have only very recently moved into the area and must wait for a period of time before they are eligible to join the waiting list. Bradshaw believes that waiting lists, which are relied on heavily by both Local Authorities and Health Authorities as a measure of need, are often inadequate. Difficulties with hospital waiting lists as a measure of expressed need or demand have been described by a number of commentators in the field of health care (see for example, Stevens & Gabbay 1991, Nottingham Health Authority 1993).

**Comparative need.** In Bradshaw's example, measuring comparative need would involve an investigation of the characteristics of elderly people already in Local Authority housing and then, through a sample survey, estimating the number of people in the community (not in Local Authority housing) who have similar characteristics.

Bradshaw suggests that this type of health needs assessment exercise would provide essential information to aid the Local Authority's decision-making. The research worker would be able to place different groups of elderly people on all four dimensions of need. For example, she would be able to say to the decision-makers that there are some elderly people who live in houses lacking basic amenities, who want to move, but are not on the waiting list, yet have similar characteristics to others residents who are already in Local Authority accommodation. By contrast, she could point out that there are other elderly people whose housing is also judged unsatisfactory by Local Authority standards, who are on the waiting list, yet who are not in need when compared to others living in Local Authority accommodation, but who want to move. The Local Authority must still make difficult decisions about which category of need, or which combination of needs, should be given priority. However, Bradshaw suggests that this kind of needs assessment exercise can clarify a Local Authority's decisions.

## Doyal and Gough: the objective basis of the concept of need

Most academic commentators believe that 'need' is a relative and subjective concept (Bradshaw 1972b, Richardson 1994). There are no such things as 'objective' needs. Rather there are simply different definitions of need held by different groups in society. One group's definition of need is no more objective than another's. It is argued that needs are not only subjective, they are also relative to a particular time and place. For example, needs in the 1990s are different from needs in the 1970s, and people living in Britain have different needs to people living in Third World countries.

Doyal and Gough's work represents an important exception to the prevailing view that needs are relative and subjective (Doyal & Gough 1992, Gough 1992, Doyal 1993). Doyal and Gough believe there to be objective needs which are common to everyone – they are universal.

Doyal and Gough's position rests on the idea that the ultimate goal of all human beings is to be able to participate fully in society (see Ch. 3). In order to be able to participate fully in society, two 'basic needs' must be met: the need for physical health, and the need for autonomy. The needs for health and autonomy, Doyal and Gough claim, are the two universal needs of all human beings. They are objective needs. They are not relative to a particular historical era or to a particular country, and they are not subjective value-judgements. Moreover, Doyal and Gough maintain, there is a moral imperative to meet fundamental human needs. The two basic needs for health and autonomy are not only the pre-requisites for participation in society, they are fundamental *rights* of all human beings (Doyal & Gough 1992).

Doyal and Gough's conceptualization of 'need' rests on the idea that there are different levels of need. There exists not only the two 'basic' needs for health and autonomy, but also a number of 'intermediate needs' which must be satisfied if the two basic needs are to be protected or improved. Intermediate needs, Doyal and Gough claim, are also universal and objective. Doyal and Gough list eleven such intermediate needs (Gough 1992):

Adequate nutritional food and water
Adequate protective housing
A non-hazardous work environment
A non-hazardous physical environment
Appropriate health care
Security in childhood
Significant primary relationships
Physical security
Economic security
Safe birth control and child-bearing
Basic education.

Doyal and Gough argue that basic and intermediate needs can be met in an almost infinite variety of ways. Thus while basic and intermediate needs are universal, ways of meeting them vary widely. Needs are met differently in different societies, and there are different services to meet need in the 1990s than existed 50 years ago. This does not mean, however, that it is not possible to compare one society's way of meeting need with another's. Doyal and Gough suggest that evaluation of the range of different policies and services to meet need should take place against the yardstick of how well they meet basic and intermediate needs. In other words, needs assessment is a process of assessing how well people's basic and intermediate needs are being met. This is in contrast to the relativists who assert that because needs, as well as ways of meeting them, differ in different societies, and differ according to who is defining them, there is no objective yardstick to assess whether one way of meeting need is better or worse than another.

Doyal and Gough stress the *non-substitutability* of need. They stress that in measuring and meeting intermediate needs, one domain of need-satisfaction cannot be traded off against another. No amount of childhood security can compensate for lack of shelter, and better nutrition cannot offset a dangerously polluted environment (Doyal & Gough 1992).

Doyal and Gough summarize their argument thus (Gough 1992):

> Though basic and intermediate needs are universal, the forms in which they can be met, and the levels at which they can be satisfied, are continually open to improvement. Yet this does not endorse a relativist position of 'anything goes'. The test of what to include, or what measures to use, or what policies to back, is always the idea of universal human need outlined above, and an acceptance that we can learn about, and judge between, better and worse methods of meeting needs....

Doyal and Gough recognize that their approach raises problems. First, it raises the question of what standard or level of need satisfaction should be set in order to calculate shortfalls in the actual level achieved? One possible solution to this problem is to set some kind of basic minimum standard, such as a 'poverty line', or a basic minimum standard of health below which people are prevented from participating in society. Doyal and Gough do not adopt this solution. They argue that shortfalls should be calculated against an optimal level rather than a minimal level (Doyal & Gough 1992). In other words, the level of need-satisfaction found in one particular locality should be judged against the yardstick of the best level that has been achieved in the wider society.

Second, Doyal and Gough recognize there are problems in answering the question of who is to decide whether or not a given policy is meeting basic and intermediate needs. One approach outlined by Doyal and Gough is the 'expert knows best' approach. (This approach corresponds with Bradshaw's concept of normative need.) For example, a doctor's, or a nutritionalist's, specialized knowledge enables them to judge people's state of health, or their dietary status, in a more informed way than can people themselves. But there are dangers in a 'top down' or normative approach. Experts and professionals are in a position of power and can put their own interests before their clients'. They may also be out of touch with the reality of ordinary people's lives, so that their proposals may be counter-productive or 'just plain stupid' (Gough 1992).

The opposite approach stresses the right of different individuals and communities to decide on their own needs. This 'community development' approach taps the detailed knowledge people have of their own communities and encourages participation and empowerment. It is this approach which underpins theories which emphasize the importance of citizenship and the ability to participate in society's policy-making processes. The drawback of this 'bottom up' approach, Doyal and Gough suggest, is that it can advantage those who already have greater privileges and resources. Most importantly, asking people to decide themselves what their needs are offers no way of reconciling competing views. All that might result from such an exercise is the lowest common denominator of whatever separate groups of people can agree on (Gough 1992).

Doyal and Gough argue that we must seek some way of overcoming the contradictions between top-down approaches which draw on 'codified' knowledge (i.e. data contained in official sources such as mortality and morbidity statistics), and bottom-up approaches relying on 'experientially grounded' knowledge. They suggest that experts and ordinary people should be enabled to confront one another in order to reconcile differences in their approaches.

### The practical application of Doyal and Gough's approach
The theoretical model outlined by Doyal and Gough served as a basis for an audit undertaken in Leeds in the early 1990s, which profiled in a comprehensive manner the needs of the population of one electoral ward, Kirkstall, which is a deprived area of Leeds (Percy-Smith & Sanderson 1992). The audit used 'codified knowledge' available in official data sources to chart local patterns of health, economic security and other indicators of need satisfaction. The audit also drew on the 'experiential knowledge' of a range of local representatives of the

community, service providers and professionals who were questioned to elicit their views about what needs existed, how far needs were being met, and what were the shortfalls in existing provision in the area. The audit also attempted to tap the views and knowledge of 'ordinary' people through a postal questionnaire and follow up interviews of a smaller sample. Finally, public meetings were arranged at which top-down and bottom-up perspectives were brought together, conflicts of opinion identified, and attempts made to resolve conflicts of opinion (Gough 1992, Percy-Smith & Sanderson 1992).

The 'Leeds audit' was successful in using 'official' data to determine, for example, levels of morbidity, mortality, and the extent of unemployment. It was also successful in soliciting the views of both professionals and lay people about which types of basic and intermediate need each group viewed as the most important, and about which policies and services each group viewed as best meeting need. For example, in looking at the needs of carers, the Leeds audit found that carers themselves stressed the importance of the provision of extra money, advice and information. Carers valued those services and policies which best met these needs. Professionals, on the other hand, emphasized respite care and holidays, which came relatively low down on carers' own list of needs (Percy-Smith & Sanderson 1992). The Leeds audit was thus able to highlight the differing perspectives of different groups in the community. The Leeds audit also provided a detailed account of the many shortcomings of current service provision, thereby documenting levels of need-satisfaction which were below the optimal level. Finally, many helpful recommendations to improve services were also made.

Those who undertook the Leeds audit acknowledged that this kind of audit, or profiling exercise, is limited in scope. Profiling, or auditing, does not provide a solution to the question of how best to distribute resources to meet need. The strength of the Leeds audit, like many similar profiling exercises carried out by nurses, was that it provided detailed and comprehensive information, including both top-down and bottom-up information, which is essential to policy makers if services are to be appropriate in meeting people's basic and intermediate needs. Those who undertook the audit believed that such an exercise can contribute to greater involvement of local people in political decision-making, but they were aware that auditing is not in itself a substitute for political decision-making. Needs auditing does not provide 'ready-made answers to the question of who gets what, how and when' (Percy-Smith & Sanderson 1992).

## Summary

The strength of Doyal and Gough's theoretical approach is that it both provides legitimacy, and suggests a particular type of methodological framework, for the kinds of auditing or profiling exercises which are currently carried out by many groups, including nurses. Doyal and Gough, in common with most practising nurses, believe that human needs cannot be 'argued away'. Doyal and Gough believe that there exist real, objective, human needs, and that it is an important and legitimate first step in meeting needs to assess levels of need-satisfaction, drawing on both top-down and bottom-up sources of information.

A further strength of Doyal and Gough's approach is the idea that the level of need-satisfaction found in a deprived area such as Kirkstall in Leeds should be judged not against some minimum acceptable standard but against the best standard achieved elsewhere. This is the idea that those whose level of need-satisfaction is furthest away from the optimal level should have a correspondingly greater share of resources targetted towards them. However, this approach can be criticized on the grounds that it raises unrealistically high expectations. Resource limitations frequently do not permit the raising of standards in deprived areas to the highest level achieved elsewhere.

The weakness of Doyal and Gough's model is that it does not provide a solution to the fact that different groups in society have different ideas about what their most important needs are, and about what are the most important policies and services to meet need. As we saw above, the Leeds audit found that in looking at the needs of carers, professionals' views of the needs of carers were out of line with carers' own perceptions. Ultimately, Doyal and Gough's theoretical position does not provide a basis for choosing between different domains of need satisfaction, or for reconciling top-down and bottom-up notions of need. This difficulty in Doyal and Gough's theoretical model was apparent when applied to the practical task of assessing needs in Kirkstall. Although the 'Leeds audit' was able to elicit the views of both professionals and lay people, there was no 'outside' criterion for reconciling different viewpoints. Doyal and Gough do not have a formula for judging between differing viewpoints (nor does anyone else) and the Leeds audit was ultimately confined to simply describing differences between the views of experts and lay people with no way of determining whose views, or whose priorities, should carry more weight.

## Economists and 'need': needs cannot all be met

Economists' views are in many respects diametrically opposed to Doyal and Gough's. Some economists take exception to the very use of the term 'need'. They believe it to be an emotive word used sometimes deliberately to 'confuse the listener and to stifle rational thought and debate' (Mooney 1992). Mooney, a health economist, points to the way in which people say things like 'We *need* a new hospital', as if this statement was somehow self-evident justification for a new hospital (Mooney 1992). Economists are relativists who do not believe there to be objective needs, and who do not believe that people have any kind of moral right to have their needs satisfied. They dismiss such beliefs as emotional and unhelpful. Economists such as Mooney and Culyer accept, however, that the term 'need' is here to stay (Culyer 1993):

> Despite its frequent use in an ill-defined way – often barely cloaking special pleading – the term (need) seems irremovable from public, political, and philosophical discussion and, consequently, on the 'if you can't beat 'em, join 'em' principle (but only on *my* terms!), it becomes necessary – stick though it may in the gullets of many economists so to do – to provide the word with suitable content.

Economists prefer to talk of 'wants', 'demands' and 'preferences' rather than 'need'. In avoiding the use of the term 'need', they are not only rejecting the emotive overtones of the term; they are also arguing that it is not for others to decide what an individual needs. To economists then, the word need is equivalent to Bradshaw's concept of normative need, and what Doyal and Gough refer to as 'top down' definitions of needs – needs as adjudged by an expert or professional. In many contexts outside the field of health-care economists would argue that it is only individual consumers who can decide what they want and what they are going to demand. It is individuals themselves and not experts or professionals who are best placed to make the appropriate judgements. This is the principle of 'consumer sovereignty', the idea that consumers should be the ones who decide what to demand. But many economists, including Mooney, accept that in the context of health-care the concepts of want, preference and demand are not sufficient, and must be supplemented by the notion of need. This is because consumers do not always have full information regarding their health status and the availability of services so that an elite body, such as the medical or nursing profession, is sometimes in a better position than individuals to decide what individuals' needs are (Mooney 1992). However, although it is sometimes necessary and acceptable that doctors or nurses determine need, Mooney (1992) maintains that consumer demand still has an important role to play: '... need does creep in but seldom if ever to the complete exclusion of demand'.

The main contribution of health economists to the 'needs debate' has been to emphasize that health care needs tend to expand over time, and this increases the cost of health-care provision. Economists stress that it is not possible to meet these ever-expanding needs. For example, before the advent of renal dialysis or kidney transplantation, end-stage renal failure often led, tragically and cheaply, to premature death (Black 1994). Today, there are many people who could benefit from transplantation or dialysis, but if scarce resources are used to offer such treatments to all those who could benefit from them, these resources cannot be used for treating others with different conditions. Given that resources are scarce health economists stress that needs must be ranked in order of priority, and difficult choices made between fulfilling one need rather than another.

Economists take issue with non-economic, 'romantic' approaches which fail to face the fact that resources are scarce so that, inevitably, not all health care needs can be met. In contrast to Doyal and Gough who stress that trade-offs cannot be made between different domains of need, Mooney stresses that there has to be a ranking of needs, and difficult decisions made about meeting one need rather than another. The ranking or prioritizing of needs has to be done, and the 'morality' of so doing must be recognized. Mooney (1992) quotes Culyer (1976) approvingly: 'we must of necessity choose from among those moral things we think we ought to do in order to devise the best 'package' in light of what is possible. Of necessity, this requires us to trade-off one need against the other. Not only ... do we do this trading off, but it is logically inescapable and, ethically, completely legitimate'.

For economists, difficult decisions about which needs to meet and how best to meet them involve comparing the costs of interventions with their benefits, and weighing up the relative costs and benefits of competing interventions. Economists' particular contribution is thus to stress that the extent to which a need will be met depends on the costs and benefits of meeting it (Mooney 1992). This is discussed further in Chapters 4, 7 and 8.

## Economists and health needs assessment

Economists do not undertake 'needs assessment' exercises and many economists are highly sceptical of needs assessment as an essential first step in deciding how to allocate health-care resources. They believe that comparisons of the costs and benefits of different health-care interventions, rather than profiles of the community's health needs, are the most appropriate first step in meeting need. Economists such as Mooney believe that needs assessment exercises of the type carried out by purchasing organizations such as District Health Authorities are very often simply misguided information-gathering exercises, the purpose of which is to evade difficult decisions about priorities. (See Ch. 10 for a description of the way in which Health Authorities assess needs.) While professing to have some sympathy for those individuals engaged in needs assessment in purchasing organizations, Mooney is nevertheless ruthless in his attack on their approach (Mooney 1994, p. 39):

> One of the potentially great advantages for needs assessors is that while they are engaged in such (needs assessment) exercises, they do not have to face up to the difficult and demanding choices involved in priority setting of services: which services to expand and, more difficult, which services to cut? Which patient to refuse? Which patients to deny life to? Caught up in the apparently laudable task of assessing needs, the key choice that is required is what data to collect. This is not to mock the needs assessors. They are human and making difficult, potentially tragic, choices . . . . . It is easy for the economist who does not have to make the choices to promote the merits of explicit rational choice. For the decision makers such choices can raise difficult moral issues . . . .

Mooney thus argues that 'needs assessment' of the type undertaken by Health Authorities should not be divorced from the questions of priority-setting and rationing. Health Authorities should not confine their activities to gathering information about health needs, they must also make difficult moral decisions about whether to meet one need or another.

To conclude: economists' most important contribution to the 'needs' debate is their insistence that meeting needs costs money, and hence the relative costs of meeting different needs must be investigated. Economists stress that needs have to be ranked in order of priority, and difficult decisions about meeting one need rather than another must be made. The economic approach is considered in more depth in Chapter 7.

## CONCLUSION

In this chapter we have explored different definitions of health needs assessment and some of the basic theories and concepts underpinning different approaches to health needs assessment. In subsequent chapters we re-visit many of the issues raised in this chapter. In the following chapter we look at some of the theoretical questions involved in defining and measuring health needs.

# Defining and measuring health

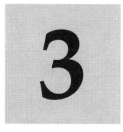

3

■ CONTENTS

## INTRODUCTION

In the previous chapter we saw that one way of defining health needs assessment is a process of measuring a particular health problem in the population. While we drew attention to some of the limitations of this definition, nevertheless a great deal of the practice of health needs assessment relies upon this definition. Much health needs assessment involves the construction of health profiles which measure the incidence and prevalence of health problems in society. In this chapter we look at some of the issues of definition and measurement involved in constructing a health profile.

The construction of a health profile relies on two sorts of information. First it relies on information about the health status of the population. This, in turn, depends on what definition of health is employed. Second it relies on information about the factors which affect health status. In this chapter we begin by looking at ways in which health and ill-health are defined and measured. We then go on to look at ways in which socio-economic factors which affect health are defined and measured through various indices of socio-economic inequality or deprivation. The chapter also identifies the main sources of data about health and about socio-economic inequalities.

## DEFINING HEALTH

Health is an elusive concept. It is often defined negatively, as the absence of disease, rather than in a positive way. It is easier to define the elements of ill-health, which might include not only disease but also pain, infirmity, disability and mental impairment, than it is to capture the elements of positive health. Moreover, it is easier to identify some of the determinants of health, such as adequate nutrition and a safe environment, than to define health itself.

Defined negatively, health is the absence of ill-health or the ability to function normally from a biological standpoint. Such negative definitions are sometimes criticized as too narrow and conservative. It is argued that there is more to life than simply being alive and being able to function properly in a biological sense. This is certainly true. On the other hand, in order to derive more from life it is necessary to survive and not to be so greatly incapacitated by illness that there can be no more to life than the suffering imposed by ill-health.

Positive definitions of health usually include both negative elements (the absence of disease) and positive elements. There is no one agreed definition of positive health. Health is sometimes defined as the ability to participate fully in life, and ill-health as those conditions which restrict people from exercising such autonomy. This is the idea expressed in the following definition, coined by Nottingham's Director of Public Health (Nottingham Health Authority 1990): '. . . . (health is) an equilibrium in which the individual is not restricted by physical or mental impairment from participating as fully as they would wish in all that their environment has to offer, or from bringing about environmental change'.

Positive health has also been defined as the ability to cope with stress, the maintenance of a strong social-support network, or a sense of well-being (Bowling 1992). The most famous example of a positive conception of health is the World Health Organization's conception of health as 'a state of complete physical, mental and social well-being, and not merely the absence of disease or infirmity' (WHO 1994). The strength of this definition is that it draws attention to the psychological and social, as well as the physical, aspects of health. However, there are difficulties with it. In the first place it is questionable whether a subjective sense of well-being is really indicative of a state of health. Drugs such as heroin can induce a sense of mental well-being (Downie et al 1994). A sense of well-being may also be associated with a high blood glucose level. Some young diabetics are known to keep their blood sugar levels high in order to avoid the unpleasant sensations and effects of hypoglycaemia, even though the long-term consequence may be harmful (Robinson et al 1995). Some psychiatric states are also accompanied by a subjective sense of euphoria, which cannot be described as true well-being (Downie et al 1994).

Another difficulty with the WHO definition is its implied breadth. There are many things aside from illness or disease which prevent us from achieving a state of complete well-being. Poverty, unemployment, oppressive cultural norms and family relations, oppressive political regimes and war can all diminish 'well-being'. Although it is important to recognize that poverty or an oppressive political regime can result in ill-health, we cannot agree with the implication of the WHO's definition that the achievement of health is the same thing as the complete eradication of all social ills. Social, economic and political deprivations *affect* health, but they do not *constitute* poor health. Although laudable in its aims the WHO's definition of health is too wide. Such an idealistic theory is unrealistic and impractical, striving towards a utopian state which it is not possible to achieve (Seedhouse 1994).

As Doyal and Gough point out, the WHO definition of health is frequently quoted and just as frequently ignored (Doyal & Gough 1992). This is because 'well-being' is so difficult to define and measure in any meaningful way. People's sense of well-being is shaped by their expectations in life, and expectations in turn vary according to the circumstances of people's lives. Sen (1985, 1992) brings this point home to us in a forcible way. Although Sen's concern is not specifically with health, but rather with welfare in general, this does not alter his argument. Sen argues that equating welfare (including health) with 'well-being' ignores all the ways in which deprived people in society lower their expectations for complete well-being and instead reconcile themselves to their fate:

> A person who has had a life of misfortune, with very little opportunities and rather little hope, may be more easily reconciled to deprivations than others reared in more fortunate and affluent circumstances . . . . . . (Sen 1985, pp. 21–22)

> The destitute thrown into beggary, the vulnerable landless labourer precariously surviving at the edge of subsistence, the over-worked domestic servant working round the clock, the subdued and subjugated housewife reconciled to her role and her fate, all tend to come to terms with their respective predicaments. The deprivations are suppressed and muffled in the necessity of endurance in uneventful survival . . . . . (Sen 1992, p. 45)

Sen thus argues that using people's own perceptions of their well-being as a yardstick of their health and welfare will distort great differences between affluent and deprived peoples. The latter lack hopes and expectations. If they do not express a sense of loss of well-being then Sen argues that it would be deeply mistaken to suggest that their lives are not lacking in important ways (Sen 1992).

Sen is not arguing that we should abandon any attempt to define and measure positive health and welfare. He is arguing rather against too superficial a definition of health and welfare as happiness, or satisfaction, or desire-fulfilment. Sen is also not arguing against the use of subjective assessments of their health by lay people. He rejects such indicators as a sense of happiness or desire-fulfilment not because they are subjective but because simply finding out whether people are happy or not is not in his view, an adequate indicator of their health or welfare. Sen's ideas have important implications for health needs assessment. As we saw in the previous chapter, and will see in subsequent chapters, many commentators believe that it is vital to consult lay people about their own health and about what services they believe are best meeting their own health needs. Sen is arguing that health needs assessment involves more than this. Like Doyal & Gough (1992) he believes that relying only on people's subjective views is not a sufficient basis for determining how successfully we are meeting need.

Both the WHO definition and that of Nottingham's Director of Public Health view health not as an end in itself but as means of achieving an utlimate goal – be it 'well-being' or autonomous social participation. Doyal & Gough (1992) get around the problem that such goals are associated with more than health by drawing a distinction between physical health and autonomy. Doyal and Gough argue that we need *both* physical health *and* autonomy to achieve full participation in life. Physical health Doyal and Gough define negatively as the minimization of death, disability and disease. Autonomy they define negatively, too, as the minimization of restrictions on people's opportunities to participate fully in life. Such restrictions include mental disorders and cognitive deprivation (such as poor language and literacy skills). Other restrictions arise from poverty and unemployment, or from oppressive cultural norms and regimes. Doyal and Gough's definition is negative in the sense that it defines physical health as the minimization of disease; and autonomy as the minimization of restrictions on opportunities. However, these two elements of their definition, Doyal and Gough suggest, add up to a positive conception. Health and autonomy are the conditions of full social participation (Doyal & Gough 1992).

In summary, health can be defined negatively as the absence of disease or more positively as encompassing more than the absence of disease. Positive definitions of health as well-being can be too superficial, providing a poor foundation for measuring health. Definitions of positive health as full participation in life suffer the drawback that participation is dependent on many factors other than health.

## MEASURING HEALTH

### Mortality

Paradoxically it is mortality or death rates which are the most commonly used measure of health. For example, *Inequalities in Health* (the *Black Report*) (Townsend & Davidson 1992) relied almost exclusively on mortality rates, as we shall see in Chapter 5. Mortality rates are used in much research as proxy measures of illness (morbidity) rates. The assumption is that if rates of premature death are high, then rates of illness are also high. This assumption was borne out in a study in the north of England by Townsend et al which found that death rates in an area were strongly associated with permanent sickness or disability, and also a high incidence of low birth weight (British Medical Association 1987, Townsend et al 1988). However, there are difficulties in relying solely on mortality rates as indicators of ill-health. There is much ill-health which does not lead to death and hence is not reflected in mortality rates. For example, many chronic and disabling conditions, such as arthritis, do not lead to premature death but cause a great deal of suffering and loss of independence. Many mental disorders too cause suffering and place severe restrictions on people's capacity to participate fully in life, yet premature death is the outcome of only a small proportion of mental disorders (British Medical Association 1987). Thus because mortality rates fail to reflect the full extent of illness, they obscure from view many important health problems which do not result in death.

The limitations of relying solely on mortality rates are universally acknowledged. However, mortality rates have positive attributes. Death is, at least, unequivocally defined, and it is universally recorded through the requirements of statutory procedures. A copy of the death registration of everyone who dies is sent to the Director of Public Health in every Health Authority (Pickin & St Leger 1994). Mortality rates thus have the advantage that they are available, objective, and unequivocal (Carstairs 1994). Thus the drawback that mortality rates fail to reflect much morbidity has to be balanced against the counter-claim that at least to the extent that mortality rates do reflect some morbidity, they do so in an objective way. It is because death rates provide a complete data base with relatively accurate descriptions of the cause of death of individual cases that many studies, including the *Black Report* (Townsend & Davidson 1992) rely heavily on this indicator.

The main source of mortality statistics is the Office of Population Censuses and Surveys (OPCS) including Series DH1 Numbers 6 (Childhood); 18 (Injury and Poisoning); 19 (Area); 20 (Cause); 26 (Perinatal and Infant); 27 (General).

## Morbidity

Most people would concur that if we wish to know the full extent of ill-health it is best to measure morbidity directly, using valid, reliable and comprehensive measures, rather than using mortality as an (inaccurate) guide to the extent of morbidity. However, this is easier said than done. Much of the data is simply not available. Consultation and treatment rates, which are recorded in activity analyses, hospital in-patient enquiries, and national studies of morbidity from general practice, provide some information about the extent of illness (British Medical Association 1987; Pickin & St Leger 1994). However, this information is limited for the purposes of gauging the extent of many illnesses because not everyone who is ill will be admitted to hospital, and many episodes of illness do not even come to the attention of the GP. Nevertheless, data such as hospital admission rates can give some indication of the extent of ill health in different geographical areas (Fig. 3.1).

Other sources of information about illness are the *Communicable Disease Report* which contains data about notifiable infectious diseases, and the *Cancer Registry*, which contains data about the incidence of the major cancers (Pickin & St Leger 1994). OPCS also

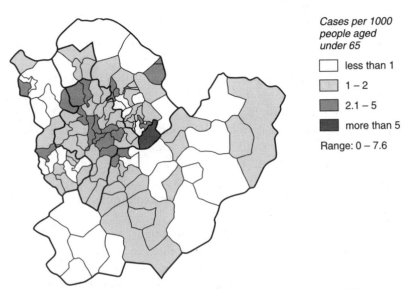

**Fig. 3.1**   Nottingham Health Authority hospital admission rate for mental illness in people aged under 65. Based on 1990 data (Reproduced with permission from Davies L 1991 Annual Report of the Director of Public Health 1991, Nottingham Health Authority).

publishes Congenital Malformation Statistics (Series MB3); Morbidity Statistics from General Practice (Series MB5); and Abortion Statistics (Series AB). Key Population and Vital Statistics for Local and Health Authority Areas are available in OPCS Series VS PP1. Further sources are the Central Statistical Office Guide to Official Statistics (published by HMSO) and *A Guide to Health Service Statistics* (Padden 1993).

## Subjective measures of health

Much chronic illness and disability is not objectively measurable, so that reliance on objective measures, based on a negative definition of health, may fail fully to reflect the extent of morbidity. In measuring both positive and negative health, it is generally felt to be important to take into account lay people's own subjective measures of their health. An important source of information which relies on such measures is *The General Household Survey* (GHS). The GHS is a continuous survey which has been running since 1971 and is based each year on a sample of the general population resident in private households in Great Britain. It takes into account people's views about the nature and degree of severity of their own ill-health or disability. The GHS is available from the OPCS.

## Positive measures of health

Bowling (1992) has pointed out that one drawback of relying on negative definitions and measures of health, such as mortality and morbidity rates, is that among a general population where the vast majority of people are not ill, information about illness and death tells us little about the health of 80–90% of the population. Although it is difficult to measure positive health, Pickin and St Leger suggest that such a daunting task can and should be undertaken. They suggest, for example, that measures of mental illness must be complemented by measures of mental health, and that measures of health status must include such measures as social support and community involvement (Pickin & St Leger 1994).

Measures of social health and social support are particularly important for nurses who see their contribution to positive health as an important aspect of their role. Although it is sometimes thought that it is not as important to measure nebulous things such as social or emotional support as it is to collect 'hard' data on rates of illness, this argument has little force when it is recognized that emotional support affects rates of ill-health. Goodwin, writing on the role of the health visitor in contribution to family health, points to a growing body of research which suggests that what health visitors working with young families vaguely call emotional support to mothers has significant measurable effects on child health. Even where social or emotional support does not have measurable effects on clinical health status, such support can contribute greatly to people's social and emotional health (Goodwin 1991).

## The instruments used to measure positive health

A number of measures have been devised which are based on a wider definition of health than the absence of disease alone. The following sources give an indication of the range of measures and scales of health and well-being that are available:

Blaxter (1985) discusses scales which include dimensions of disease, functional disability, 'illness' or frequent symptoms, 'malaise' or lack of psychological well being, and fitness. Bowling (1992) includes a large number of scales listed under the headings of functional ability, broader measures of health status, psychological well-being, social networks and social support, and life satisfaction and morale. Moreover, a recent WHO publication lists basic questionnaires available under the broad headings of general, physical, mental and social health (Kunst & Mackenbach 1994). It will be recalled from Chapter 1, however, that one social scientist who has been actively engaged in the assessment of chronic illness warns against using such tools uncritically or too enthusiastically (Fitzpatrick 1995). Fitzpatrick refers to a revolution in the development of a 'vast array of survey-based instruments' by social scientists in collaboration with epidemiologists. These instruments include interview schedules or questionnaires to assess 'quality of life', 'functional status', 'health profile' etc. Fitzpatrick (1995, p. 184) suggests that these instruments have in common that: '. . . they are intended as practical, economical, reliable. and valid means of obtaining aspects of patients' personal experience of symptoms and the associated physical, social and psychological sequelae of their illness'.

Fitzpatrick describes a number of potential benefits to be derived from the use of these instruments, including: richer information about subjects; the ability to distinguish between patient groups and to predict demand on health services; the improvement of health professionals' awareness of the personal and social consequences of chronic illness for their patients; the potential to assess health outcomes of health care using valid and reliable tools; and their sensitivity to the salient aspects of chronic illness. However, Fitzpatrick highlights a number of subtle difficulties associated with many of these instruments. For example, instruments which appear to cover similar dimensions of illness may, in reality, be tapping important but different phenomena. Thus one scale which purports to be measuring the social dimensions of someone's experience of disease may, in reality, be measuring something completely different to another scale which uses similar terminology. For example, 'feeling a burden' and 'infrequency of social contact' may be used respectively on different scales to measure the social dimensions of chronic disease. However, both may have different meanings and consequences for the individual concerned. Therefore, in order to interpret the results obtained from a qualitative indicator arising from the use of a particular scale, health care practitioners in daily practice would need to have detailed understanding of the *specific* dimensions measured by different scales, and this is rarely a practical possibility.

Fitzpatrick also points out that such instruments are rarely sensitive to important short- and long-term fluctuations in the severity and nature of symptoms in chronic illness. Additionally, they impose certain components of 'quality of life' in their assessments when individuals may have very different values in respect to what is important to them in the management of their condition. Fitzpatrick's major criticism is therefore that such tools not only 'smooth out' individual differences in consumer attitudes to, and management of, chronic disease but also that, in focusing 'too exclusively on the health status or quality-of-life deficits of the individual with a chronic illness', they ignore 'the impact that the social context has in shaping and determining handicaps' (Fitzpatrick 1995).

## MEASURING DEPRIVATION

Health, defined either positively and negatively, is affected by social and economic factors. Measures of such factors as low income or poor housing conditions are important because they tell us indirectly about people's health. It is a well established research finding that people who are socio-economically disadvantaged suffer a heavier burden of illness and have higher mortality rates than their better-off counterparts (Kunst & Mackenbach 1994). Thus is assessing health needs, measures of mortality, morbidity and other positive measures of health will provide some indication of the size of the health problem in a given community. However, if we wish to know also in which sub-groups of a population health problems are likely to be concentrated, then it is vital to measure socio-economic inequalities or deprivation.

Occupational class has been widely used as an indicator of socio-economic status. It is the main measure relied upon in the *Black Report* (Townsend & Davidson 1992; see also Ch. 5). Two widely used measures of occupational class are the Registrar General's classification by occupational class, and the scale of socio-economic groups which brings together people with similar skills and life-styles. In both scales people are ranked according to the occupation of the head of the household. *The Health Divide* (Townsend & Davidson 1992) observes that both scales are taken as an indication of people's socio-economic status, as a 'a rough guide to the way of life and living standards experienced by the separate groups and their families; they correlate fairly well with other components of social position, like education and income'.

*Registrar General's occupational social class*

  I   Professional (e.g. lawyer, doctor, accountant)
  II  Intermediate (e.g. teacher, nurse, manager)
IIIN  Skilled non-manual (e.g. typist, shop assistant)
IIIM  Skilled manual (e.g. miner, bus driver, cook)
 IV  Partly skilled manual (e.g. farm worker, bus conductor)
  V  Unskilled manual (e.g. cleaner, labourer)

*Socio-economic groups*

1 Professional
2 Employers and managers
3 Intermediate junior non-manual
4 Skilled manual
5 Semi-skilled manual and personal service
6 Unskilled manual

As an indicator, occupational class is not without problems. One major problem is that of classifying children, women and economically inactive people about whom such an indicator may tell us very little (Kunst & Mackenbach 1994). Unemployed and retired people are classified according to their previous occupation but this tells us little about their current social and economic position. It is known that unemployed people are at greater risk of ill-health, but this is obscured in measures which do not classify unemployed people separately (Westcott et al 1985, Moser et al 1986, Dahlgren & Whitehead 1992, Wilson & Walker 1993, Morris et al 1994). Similarly, lone mothers and their children, who are at higher risk of deprivation and poor health, are not identified (British Medical Association 1987). It is now generally agreed that occupational class is becoming a poorer measure of socio-economic status. This is because such trends as the growth in home ownership, second incomes, single parenthood and unemployment are cutting across the relationship assumed in measures of occupational class between a man's occupation and family resources (British Medical Association 1987). Despite their limitations, a great deal of the available evidence on the relationship between socio-economic status and health is based on measures of occupational class. For example, the *Black Report* (Townsend & Davidson 1992) relied heavily on occupational status. In part this is because this type of data has been the most readily available. Occupation has been recorded historically in conjunction with the statutory registration of deaths and, as a result, it has been possible to draw on a comprehensive data base, and to compare death rates in different occupational groups over time.

Measures of socio-economic status such as the Registrar General's classification by occupation are used to rank individuals on a scale. In recent years alternative scales have been developed which rank small areas rather than individuals on an index of deprivation. There exist currently a plethora of measures of deprivation based on a composite of demographic, social and material indicators. Many of these indicators are based on information provided by the Census and are available from the OPCS.

Examples of commonly used composite measures of deprivation

**Table 3.1** Some commonly used composite measures of deprivation

| Jarman index | Nottinghamshire County Council |
|---|---|
| | *Low income* |
| % Elderly living alone | % Households with no car |
| % Aged under 5 | % Households children receiving free |
| % Social class V | school meals |
| % Unemployed | % Households including a lone parent |
| % One-parent families | % Persons dependent on those in |
| % In overcrowded households | employment |
| % Changed address within | |
| 1 year | *Unemployment* |
| % Ethnic minorities | % Adults unemployed |
| | % Youths unemployed |
| | |
| | *Poor housing* |
| | % Households > one person per room |
| | % Households lacking central heating |
| | |
| | *Poor health* |
| | % Persons with limiting long-term illness |
| | % Low-weight babies |
| | |
| | *Family difficulties* |
| | % Youths taken into Local Authority care |
| | % Youths in trouble with the police |
| | |
| | *Educational difficulties* |
| | % Youths leaving school at 16 |
| | |
| | *Lack of skills* |
| | % Semi-skilled workers |
| | % Un-skilled workers |

are the Jarman index, the Carstairs index, the Townsend index, Department of the Environment index, and Nottinghamshire County Council's index, all of which combine several indicators of deprivation. For example, Table 3.1 compares the Jarman and Nottinghamshire County Council indices.

The various indices of deprivation all differ in the indicators they include, and there are therefore differences in their ranking of different areas as deprived. For example, the Department of the Environment index places the ten most deprived Local Authorities in the country in London, whereas the use of a different index, such as the Townsend index, will rank some Local Authorities in the North of England amongst the most deprived (British Medical Association 1987). There is also a problem of comparison when different authorities, such as Health Authorities and Local Authorities, use a different geographical base in addition to a different index of deprivation. For example, Figure 3.2 shows Townsend Deprivation scores for every electoral ward within Nottingham Health Authority. By contrast Figure 3.3 shows levels of 'social need' rather than 'deprivation' for different census enumeration districts in the Greater Nottingham area.

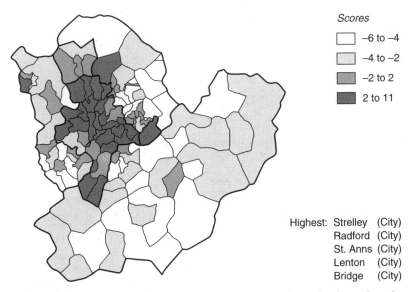

Scores

☐ −6 to −4

☐ −4 to −2

▨ −2 to 2

■ 2 to 11

Highest:  Strelley  (City)
          Radford   (City)
          St. Anns  (City)
          Lenton    (City)
          Bridge    (City)

**Fig. 3.2**  Nottingham Health District Townsend Deprivation Scores by electoral ward (Reproduced with permission from Davies L 1993 Annual Report of the Director of Public Health 1993, Nottingham Health Authority).

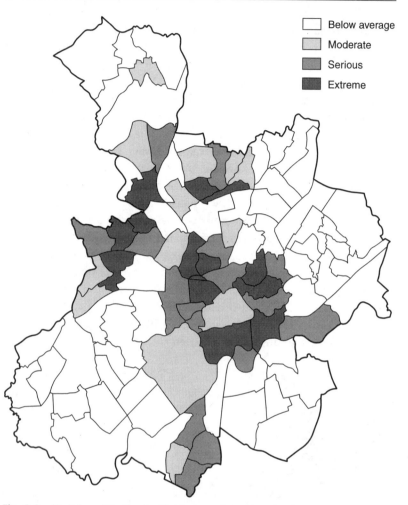

**Fig. 3.3** 'Social need' in Greater Nottingham (Reproduced with permission from Nottinghamshire County Council (1994)).

Would-be health needs assessors need to recognise that different measures of deprivation, and differences in the populations to which they are applied, reflect different purposes, so that confusion can result if an attempt is made to make direct comparisons between data gathered for different purposes.

Some of the indicators used in measures of deprivation are direct measures of deprivation. For example, 'unemployment' is a comparatively direct measure of deprivation. Other indicators are less direct, they are proxy measures. For example, 'not owning a car' is an indirect indicator, or proxy, of low income or a low standard of living (Nottinghamshire Structure Plan 1983; Kunst & Mackenbach 1994). Other indicators are measures of groups at risk of deprivation, rather than measures of deprivation itself. For example 'membership of an ethnic minority group' is an indicator of the risk of experiencing deprivation.

## Problems with measures of deprivation

### Validity

One important problem with deprivation measures is that of validity. Validity is concerned with whether or not an indicator actually measures the underlying attribute which it purports to measure (Bowling 1992). For example, it can be questioned whether 'overcrowding' is captured by a measure of 'proportion of people living at a density of more than two persons per room' (Doyal & Gough 1992).

It was the problem of validity which led Jarman to omit one of his original indicators. Initially the Jarman index was made up of ten variables but subsequently two variables were omitted. One of these was 'households lacking basic amenities' which was measured by whether a household had exclusive use of a bath and an inside WC. Because the regulations for council houses require these basic amenities to be present, poor council housing estates appeared good on this 'lacking basic amenities' variable, even though they lacked amenities other than these very basic ones, and even though they showed up as bad on the 'overcrowding' variable. Thus the 'lacking basic amenities' variable was not valid. It did not capture the poor housing conditions that it was designed to capture, and it was therefore discarded (Jarman 1984).

### Lack of an appropriate indicator

Since it is not always possible to measure deprivation directly, proxy measures must be found; there must be some way of linking what we want to measure to what it is practically possible to measure. However, sometimes it is just not possible to find a satisfactory indicator.

### Sources of information

Most measures of deprivation rely heavily on the census as a source of information, so that the construction of deprivation measures is constrained by what information is available from the census. The

Jarman index confined itself exclusively to census information. Where variables are included in deprivation measures which are not census variables there may be difficulties in obtaining data. Originally, Jarman considered using 'crime rate' as an indicator of deprivation, but this was not a census variable. However, in this instance the problem was not insurmountable. Jarman was aware of a survey undertaken by the Royal College of General Practitioners which showed a high correlation between 'crime rate' and 'overcrowding'. Since Jarman was including overcrowding as an indicator, the omission of crime rate was felt not to be too grave (Jarman 1983).

The major drawback of the census is that it is only carried out at 10-yearly intervals so that the further away we move in time from the most recent census, the more out-of-date is the census information. However, for some kinds of information there are other sources. For example, the Department of Employment produces counts of the number of persons unemployed for every quarter (NOMIS data) (Jarman & Bajekal 1994).

## Choosing a cut-off point

The selection of a cut-off score above which a population is defined as deprived and below which it is defined as not deprived is obviously arbitrary to an extent (Jarman 1983). The Nottinghamshire Deprived Area Study (Nottinghamshire Structure Plan 1983) classified areas (zones) according to whether they were suffering 'extreme' disadvantage (a score above 20); 'serious' disadvantage (above 10); or 'moderate' disadvantage (a score above 5.32 which was the average of scores for all zones). Clearly, these cut-off points are arbitrary to a degree; other cut-off points could have been chosen.

## Comparing different levels of population

A focus of analysis on very large populations sometimes masks differences between the smaller populations of which the larger population is made up. For example, when electoral wards are merged into districts, the best and worst wards tend to cancel each other out, and hence differences between districts may not be as wide as those between electoral wards. Similarly when districts are merged into regions, the differences between districts are cancelled out in a similar way (Irving 1985).

## The 'ecological fallacy'

The British Medical Association suggests that there are good reasons for measuring deprivation on an area basis rather than on an individual basis because most planning of health and social services is conducted on an area basis and therefore requires area-based information about deprivation and health (British Medical Association 1987). However, it is important to recognize that not everybody who lives in a deprived area is deprived and, conversely, that some deprived people live in affluent areas (British Medical Association 1987).

The main problem with area based studies (often referred to as 'ecological' studies) is what is known as the ecological fallacy. This is the problem of inferring that an association which holds true at one level of population analysis also holds true for much smaller populations, or for individual people (Gilman et al 1994). For example, at an area level it may appear that there is an association between housing tenure and health, with owner-occupation being associated with better health than council-house dwelling. However, analysis at the smaller population level may show that there is no such association. For some smaller communities or individual families, living in a council house might be associated with better health than owner occupation. It might be that council house dwellers enjoy low rents as compared to the high mortgages of some owner-occupiers, and this might enable the former to spend more on an adequate diet. Moreover, council house dwellers might be housed in a more clean and safe environment. Thus, although area level studies can provide evidence of an association in that area between various indicators of deprivation and poor health, they cannot be used to infer a relationship, for example between housing tenure or unemployment and poor health in a particular individual, family or small community within that area.

That individual families often have very different health experiences, even when suffering from the same kinds of deprivations will be a situation familiar to many community health workers. Area-based or ecological studies may fail to provide answers to questions about why families in apparently similar social and material circumstances have such differing health experiences. Health care practitioners need to be aware that these different experiences are particularly important in local health needs assessment, for a reliance on associations derived from ecological analysis can lead so easily to the stereotyping of individuals and families. Furthermore, as Klein (1991) argues, a reliance on correlations or associations found at an area level, based on no real understanding of the processes giving rise to them – and therefore no real understanding of the processes which might confound them – are a poor basis for action at all levels, from the level of national policy to interventions at the level of individual families.

## CONCLUSION

In this chapter we have introduced some ideas concerning the definition and measurement of health and deprivation in constructing a health profile. We have seen how, through measures of health status and measures such as deprivation indices, the health needs of a population can be diagnosed. In Chapters 5, 11 and 12 we look at the way in which measures of health status and deprivation have been used to profile the needs of local populations.

In the following chapter we widen our analysis by exploring central government's approach to health needs assessment. We look at the government's *Health of the Nation* strategy which sets specific outcomes or targets for improving health. We also look at government guidance to District Health Authorities for assessing local population health needs.

# Health needs assessment: the approach of central government

**4**

## INTRODUCTION

The *Health of the Nation* (Department of Health 1992) was an attempt on the part of government to assess the health needs of the nation and to set priorities and targets to improve health. In the first part of this chapter we look in depth at the government's *Health of the Nation* strategy, exploring its strengths and weaknesses as an approach to health needs assessment. In the second part of the chapter we look at government guidance to District Health Authorities for assessing the health needs of the local populations they serve.

## SUMMARY OF THE *HEALTH OF THE NATION*

The *Health of the Nation* Green Paper was published in 1991, the White Paper, July 1992 (Department of Health 1991a, 1992). The Green Paper (like all government Green Papers) was a consultation document, published in advance of the White Paper in order to consult and invite comment. The subsequent White Paper informed the public of future policy intent. It is in the Green Paper that the government's thinking is most clearly elaborated. Many of the critiques of the *Health of the Nation* discussed below relate to the Green Paper.

The aim of the Health of the Nation initiative is simple: it is to secure improvements in the health of the population of England

(Department of Health 1992). The *Health of the Nation* Green Paper (Department of Health 1991a) sets out a number of key policy objectives which underpin the entire approach; these are:

- to identify and focus on the main health problems;
- to focus as much on the promotion of good health and the prevention of disease as on treatment, care and rehabilitation, while ensuring that work on either is not at the expense of the other;
- to recognise that health is determined by a whole range of influences, from genetic inheritance, through personal behaviour, family and social circumstances to the physical and social environment so that action for the improvement of health must be spread widely from individuals to Government;
- to recognise that concerted action demands greater collaboration between those involved at national and local level, within and outside the NHS;
- to secure a proper balance between central strategic direction and local and individual discretion, flexibility and initiative;
- to secure the best possible use of available resources.

The overall aim of the *Health of the Nation* is to secure 'health gains'. This is defined to mean both increasing longevity and improving the quality of life. . . . 'adding years to life and life to years' (Department of Health 1992).

## Choosing priorities: criteria for 'key area' status

The *Health of the Nation* recognizes that a strategy for health cannot address every area of health care. There have to be priorities (Department of Health 1991a, 1992). In choosing priority areas ('key areas'), the Green Paper specified three criteria against which all possible candidates for key area status were to be judged (Department of Health 1991a, 1992). The first is the 'burden of disease' criterion:

> The area should be a major cause of premature death or avoidable ill-health (sickness and/or disability) either in the population as a whole or amongst specific groups of people (Department of Health 1991a, p. 26, para 5.4).

The second criterion is about effectiveness:

> The area should be one where effective interventions are possible, offering significant scope for improvement in health (Department of Health 1991a, p. 26, para 5.4).

The first two criteria are thus attempts to ensure that the key areas selected will be those where there is both the 'greatest need' and greatest scope for effective interventions to improve the health of the country (Department of Health 1992).

The third criterion states that:

> It should be possible to set objectives and targets in the chosen area, and monitor progress towards achievement through indicators (Department of Health 1991a, p. 26, para 5.4).

It is acknowledged that the current state of knowledge about levels of illness, and the scope for improvements, is incomplete and that indicators are lacking in many areas. For these reasons it is suggested that strict adherence to the three criteria would be unreasonable in the early stages. A 'pragmatic' approach is recommended, where targets are set in the knowledge that information and understanding is currently far from complete (Department of Health 1991a).

## The choice of key areas

Five key areas were eventually chosen, and targets for action within these key areas set. These five key areas and their associated targets are set out in the White Paper, as shown in Box 4.1.

In addition, four 'risk factor' targets were chosen; these are shown in Box 4.2.

The White Paper stressed that these key areas were not for all time. Other key areas should be included over time.

The Green Paper listed many more candidates for 'key area' status than the five which were eventually chosen. The Green Paper originally discussed 16 possibilities and many others were suggested during the consultation process (Table 4.1). In the event, nine out the range of candidates set out in the Green Paper were selected in the White Paper, five as the main key areas in which targets were to be set and four as 'risk factor' targets (see above).

It is interesting to note that two areas, cancer and HIV/AIDS, which were considered in the Green Paper not to meet the three criteria sufficiently to merit selection as key areas, were finally selected. The explanation for the final selection of cancers as key areas is relatively straightforward. Because effective treatments exist for only some types of cancer (criterion 2), it was felt that to treat cancer as a single area was inappropriate), but that to choose as target areas four

**Box 4.1** *Health of the Nation:* main targets

*Coronary heart disease and stroke*[1]

To reduce death rates for both CHD and stroke in people under 65 by at least 40% by the year 2000 (*Baseline 1990*)

To reduce the death rate for CHD in people aged 65–74 by at least 30% by the year 2000 (*Baseline 1990*)

To reduce the death rate for stroke in people aged 65–74 by at least 40% by the year 2000 (*Baseline 1990*)

*Cancers*[1]

To reduce the death rate for breast cancer in the population invited for screening by at least 25% by the year 2000 (*Baseline 1990*)

To reduce the incidence of invasive cervical cancer by at least 20% by the year 2000 (*Baseline 1986*)

To reduce the death rate for lung cancer under the age of 75 by at least 30% in men and by at least 15% in women by 2010 (*Baseline 1990*)

To halt the year-on-year increase in the incidence of skin cancer by 2005

*Mental illness*[1]

To improve significantly the health and social functioning of mentally ill people

To reduce the overall suicide rate by at least 15% by the year 2000 (*Baseline 1990*)

To reduce the suicide rate of severely mentally ill people by at least 33% by the year 2000 (*Baseline 1990*)

*HIV/AIDS and sexual health*

To reduce the incidence of gonorrhoea by at least 20% by 1995 (*Baseline 1990*), as an indicator of HIV/AIDS trends

To reduce by at least 50% the rate of conceptions amongst the under 16s by the year 2000 (*Baseline 1989*)

*Accidents*[1]

To reduce the death rate for accidents among children aged under 15 by at least 33% by 2005 (*Baseline 1990*)

To reduce the death rate for accidents among young people aged 15–24 by at least 25% by 2005 (*Baseline 1990*)

To reduce the death rate for accidents among people aged 65 and over by at least 33% by 2005 (*Baseline 1990*)

[1] The 1990 baseline for all mortality targets represents an average of the 3 years centred around 1990. See Department of Health (1992, pp 124–126) 'Technical notes on target setting and monitoring'.

---

**Box 4.2** *Health of the Nation:* risk factor targets

*Smoking*

To reduce the prevalence of cigarette smoking to no more than 20% by the year 2000 in both men and women (a reduction of a third) (*Baseline 1990*)

To reduce consumption of cigarettes by at least 40% by the year 2000 (*Baseline 1990*)

In addition to the overall reduction in prevalence, at least 33% of women smokers to stop smoking at the start of their pregnancy by the year 2000

To reduce smoking prevalence of 11–15 year olds by at least 33% by 1994 (to less than 6%) (*Baseline 1988*)

*Diet and Nutrition*

To reduce the average percentage of food energy derived by the population from saturated fatty acids by at least 35% by 2005 (to no more than 11% of food energy) (*Baseline 1990*)

To reduce the average percentage of food energy derived from total fat by the population by at least 12% by 2005 (to no more than about 35% of total food energy) (*Baseline 1990*)

To reduce the proportion of men and women aged 16–64 who are obese by at least 25% and 33% respectively by 2005 (to no more than 6% of men and 8% of women) (*Baseline 1986/87*)

To reduce the proportion of men drinking more than 21 units of alcohol per week and women drinking more than 14 units per week by 30% by 2005 (to 18% of men and 7% of women) (*Baseline 1990*)

*Blood pressure*

To reduce mean systolic blood pressure in the adult population by at least 5mm Hg by 2005 (*Baseline to be derived from new national health survey*)

*HIV/AIDS*

To reduce the percentage of injecting drug misusers who report sharing injecting equipment in the previous 4 weeks from 20% in 1990 to no more than 10% by 1997 and no more than 5% by the year 2000

---

See Department of Health (1992, pp 124–126) 'Technical notes on target setting and monitoring'.

---

separate, treatable cancers was appropriate (Department of Health 1991a). The reasons for the selection of HIV/AIDS are less straight-forward. These are discussed in the section entitled *The Process of Selecting Key Areas: the Case of HIV/AIDS,* below.

**Table 4.1** Identifying key areas: possible key areas, objectives and targets

| Area | Criterion 1 Major cause of concern | Criterion 2 Scope for improvement | Criterion 3 Ability to set targets |
|---|---|---|---|
| Coronary heart disease | Greatest single cause of premature death | Healthy living Effective treatment | Yes |
| Stroke | 12% of all deaths 5% of deaths under 65 years | Healthy living Detection and treatment of raised blood pressure Rehabilitation | Yes |
| Cancers | 25% of all deaths | Not for all cancers For some – healthy living Screening for breast and cervical cancers | Not for all cancers Screening targets for breast and cervical cancer + see smoking target |
| Smoking | Largest single preventable cause of death | Not smoking | Yes |
| Eating and drinking habits | Contribution to many aspects of health and ill-health | Healthier eating and drinking habits | Yes |
| Physical activity | Contribution to many aspects of health and ill-health | More people taking regular physical activity | Not at this stage – further information needed |
| Prevention of accidents | Most common cause of death under 30 | Improvements in engineering, design, environment etc Education, awareness Legislation and other controls | Yes |
| Health of pregnant women, infants and children | Key indicator of the nation's health | Wide subject – scope varies for different aspects | Yes |
| Diabetes | 4–5% of total health care expenditure on care of people with diabetes | Effective treatment and care | Yes |

**Table 4.1** *Cont'd*

| Area | Criterion 1 Major cause of concern | Criterion 2 Scope for improvement | Criterion 3 Ability to set targets |
|---|---|---|---|
| Mental health | 20% of total NHS expenditure | Transition to a district-based service | Yes |
| HIV/AIDS | Greatest new threat to public health this century | Safe sexual and intravenous drug using behaviour | Not at this stage – further information needed |
| Other communicable diseases | | | |
| (a) preventable by immunization | Potential for harm should immunization rates fall | Immunization | Yes |
| (b) hospital acquired infection | 10% of inpatients have an infection acquired in hospital | Good practice | Yes |
| Food safety | | | |
| (a) foodborne diseases | Cause of considerable degree of ill-health, though not many deaths Underlying rising trend in cases | Improvements in hygiene Increase in awareness Effective surveillance Regulation | Not at this stage – more needs to be known about incidence of food poisoning |
| (b) chemical safety of food | Undoubted potential for harm to human health in absence of effective measures | Continued research and assessment. Regulation and other controls | Limited ability to set targets in terms of human health |
| Rehabilitation services | Wide subject covering a variety of areas of concern | Scope for intervention varies | Yes – in specific areas |
| Asthma | Substantial morbidity – lost schooling and sickness absence | Effective treatment and care | Yes |

**Table 4.1** Cont'd

| Area | Criterion 1 Major cause of concern | Criterion 2 Scope for improvement | Criterion 3 Ability to set targets |
|------|-----------------------------------|-----------------------------------|-----------------------------------|
| Environmental quality | Potential for harm to health if standards of protection are inadequate. Unrealised potential for promotion of health and well-being when standards are sufficiently high | Improvement in abatement technologies, stricter standards which are effectively enforced mobilization of public interest | Yes – in most areas |

The government saw two constraints in implementing their strategy: *knowledge* and *resources*. Knowledge about which interventions are effective is patchy, and resources are scarce. Since resources are finite, a health strategy must take this into account by setting priorities which make the best use of those resources (Department of Health 1991a).

Finally, the Green Paper stresses once more that 'health' is not simply the product of health care services. The objectives and targets which are set are not only the responsibility of governments or health care services. Those involved in achieving them include (Department of Health 1991a):

- Individuals
- Families
- Communities
- Health care services
- Personal social services
- Health professions
- The education service
- The voluntary sector
- Industry, commerce and trades unions
- The media
- Government, central and local
- International organizations.

# THE *HEALTH OF THE NATION*: DISCUSSION

## The epidemiological versus the economic approach to setting priorities

The *Health of the Nation* is about determining priorities and setting targets on the basis of an epidemiological assessment of health needs. Important criticism of this kind of epidemiological approach to health needs assessment have been made by economists. To understand these criticisms, it is helpful to look at some of the differences between epidemiology and economics. These differences are explored in greater depth in Chapters 6 and 7.

Epidemiology's main focuses of interest are on specific health problems. Epidemiologists concentrate much of their efforts on identifying how much illness and premature death there is through descriptive studies and surveys of the incidence and prevalence of disease. Epidemiologists are also interested in how effective health care interventions are. Only if it is known what measures are effective can morbidity and premature mortality be reduced. The epidemiological approach thus attempts to determine the size of a health problem (the incidence and prevalence of an illness); and it attempts to monitor the effectiveness of health care interventions. The basic epidemiological approach does not take cost into consideration. In setting priorities, the two most important factors are the relative magnitude of the problem, and the effectiveness of interventions to treat it (Frater & Sheldon 1993).

Economists come to the question of setting priorities from a different angle. Like epidemiologists, health economists view the achievement of 'health gains' as an important goal. However, unlike epidemiologists, economists insist that the idea of measuring the size of health problems as a preliminary to trying to achieve health gains is an utterly forlorn and misguided aim. The size of the problem will always greatly outstrip the resources at our disposal to deal exhaustively with it. The fundamental question economists ask is not 'What is the size of the health problem?' It is 'How can scarce resources best be used to bring about maximum health gains?' Economists argue that if the aim is to maximize health gains, then information about the total burden of disease is not relevant (Drummond 1993). What is relevant is information about the effectiveness of interventions, and information about their costs in relation to their effectiveness or benefits. If the aim of health care is to maximize health gains, then the way to do this is not to allocate resources pro rata according to the size of the problem, but rather to measure the costs and benefits of different health care interventions and to choose that combination of health care interventions which maximizes the benefits from available resources (Donaldson 1994). Thus for economists, it is not the size of the problem which determines the share of total resources which should be allocated to it; it is the relative costs and benefits of interventions to treat different health problems that determines how resources should be allocated between different health problems. This is explained further in Chapter 7.

There is only one matter about which the economic and the epidemiological approaches are in agreement. This is that *effectiveness* is important. Both economists and epidemiologists stress that reductions in morbidity and mortality are dependent on effective health care interventions. Thus both the epidemiological and the economic approaches rely on knowledge about the effectiveness of health care interventions.

## Needs assessment, priority setting and the choice of the *Health of the Nation* criteria: the economists' critique

In his critique of the *Health of the Nation*, Mooney is highly critical of the epidemiological approach adopted (Mooney 1994). We saw in Chapter 2 that there are two epidemiological definitions of 'need'. The first is related to the extent of illness. The more illness there is in a community, the greater is 'need'. The second, more sophisticated definition of need is the 'capacity to benefit from health care'. Here, need is related to the effectiveness of interventions. The *Health of the Nation* appears to rely on both definitions. The first *Health of the Nation* criterion for key area status, that the area should be a major cause of premature death or avoidable ill-health, contains the idea that the extent of need is related to the size of the problem. The second *Health of the Nation* criterion, that effective interventions must be possible, is related to the 'need as the ability to benefit' definition.

Mooney argues that neither criterion can provide us with a means of determining priorities. In relation to the first, 'burden of disease' criterion, Mooney questions the idea implicit in much health policy that those illnesses which give rise to the biggest health problems should be given priority (Mooney 1994, pp. 37, 39):

... there does seem (to be) some sort of 'big problem' imperative in much of health policy. Yet there is little logic in the notion that simply because the disease that I suffer from happens to be a common one, that that by itself and *ceteris paribus* should mean that I get higher priority for treatment than someone suffering from a rather less common disease.

Needs assessment is based on faulty logic – the faulty logic of the imperative of the 'size of the problem'. That faulty logic needs to be exposed – and exposed again. It is so pervasive in health care. The fact that it is pervasive, however, is no reason for believing that it is in any sense right.

Mooney objects to the first *Health of the Nation* criterion because it suggests that priorities should be set on the basis of the size of a problem – whether or not the problem can be dealt with (Mooney 1994). Although the *Health of the Nation* also employs the 'effectiveness/ability to benefit' criterion, Mooney's criticism is still applicable. All small problems for which there are highly effective treatments from which peolple could benefit, do not get past the first *Health of the Nation* criterion (Mooney 1994).

The *Health of the Nation* acknowledges that resources are scarce, and that the best possible use must be made of them. Although the White Paper goes as far as to stress that in all key areas there must be 'scope for making cost-effective improvements in the overall health of the country' (Department of Health 1992), the strategy falls short of actually including cost-effectiveness as a criterion for key area status.

Mooney (1994) and other economists are critical of this failure to include cost-effectiveness as a criterion. They argue that if the best use is to be made of resources, if health gains are to be maximized, then comparative assessments of the costs of health-care interventions in relation to their benefits are essential (Akehurst et al 1991).

The *Health of the Nation* involves no weighing up of the costs and benefits of different health care interventions and economists thus reject the strategy as failing to provide a basis for choosing priorities (Mooney 1994). Mooney concludes that the *Health of the Nation* is 'sloganizing for health in the sense of saying: let's get rid of the big health problems; rather than: let's maximize the health of the nation' (Mooney 1994).

Mooney's and others' criticisms, although harsh, do have validity. For example, the *Health of the Nation* proposes that as much emphasis should be placed on the promotion of health as on the treatment of ill health while ensuring that 'work on either is not at the expense of the other' (Department of Health 1991a). Yet as the Radical Statistics Health Group, the RCN and Akehurst et al all point out, without any commitment of extra resources it is difficult to see how investment in one area is not at the expense of another (Radical Statistics Health Group 1991; Royal College of Nursing 1991a; Akehurst et al 1991). The *Health of the Nation* can thus be accused of evading difficult choices between health promotion and treatment services, and of failing to provide a basis for deciding which services to expand and which to contract within each of the two broad areas of prevention and treatment (Mooney 1994).

Mooney's attack on needs assessment stems from his economic approach. It is not necessary to know the size of the problem to arrive at priorities which maximize health gains. However, as Mooney himself concedes, assessing total needs *is* relevant when the aim is not the maximization of health gains, but rather the equitable distribution of health care resources. It is in relation to equity that the epidemiological approach has potentially much to offer and the strictly economic approach very little. However, as we shall see below, the goal of ensuring an equitable distribution of resources was not a dominant concern in the *Health of the Nation*.

## NON-ECONOMIC CRITIQUES OF THE *HEALTH OF THE NATION*

### The process of selecting key areas: the case of HIV/AIDS

Although the process by which the final key areas were selected is not discussed in either Green or White paper the final selection of HIV/AIDS when it had initially been ruled out raises questions about how the selection was made. It appears that it was possible to choose AIDS/HIV as a key area because the *Health of the Nation* allowed for the selection of key areas where knowledge – in this instance about the prevalence of HIV/AIDS – was lacking (Department of Health 1991a). However, other potential key areas such as the health of elderly people, asthma and back pain, where it was also felt that knowledge was lacking, were not included. In these latter cases, it was felt that further research and development was necessary before national targets could be set (Department of Health 1992). Second, it appears that it was possible to select AIDS/HIV because the first criterion for key area status is somewhat ambiguous. It is sometimes stated that the health problem must be 'a major cause of premature death or avoidable illness' (Department of Health 1991a) and at other times that it must be 'a major cause of concern' (see Boxes 4.1 and 4.2, pp 54–55). AIDS/HIV is certainly the latter but it is not (yet) the former in Britain.

We are not suggesting, as have others, that the final selection of key areas was 'arbitrary' (Akehurst et al 1991) or that the key areas were 'plucked out of the sky' (Smith 1991a); neither do we accept at face value the Government's own assertion that their final selection relied on 'pragmatic' considerations (Department of Health 1991a). Governments of all persuasions are apt to try to justify their decisions as 'pragmatic', common sense. The choices of key areas were *political*. They were not technical choices derived from some kind of value-neutral application of epidemiological or economic principles; neither were they arbitrary. They were political choices about what the government of the day deemed to be the most important national problems: 'A strategy for health will have succeeded if... it is judged that priority was given and energies devoted to what mattered most at the time' (Department of Health 1991a, p. 20, para 4.20).

There is nothing wrong with governments making political choices. On the contrary, political decision-making is the *raison d'etre* of government. Our point is to underline that setting priorities in health care always involves value-judgements and political decisions. Whether one draws on epidemiological or economic principles, the necessity of forming value-judgements and making political decisions cannot be avoided. Ultimately, decisions about priorities in health care are always *political* decisions.

## Equity as a criterion for key area status

The *Health of the Nation* was the government's response to the World Health Organization's European-wide initiative for achieving Health for All by the Year 2000. However, the targets set by the WHO, in stark contrast to the *Health of the Nation* targets, were very much concerned with the question of equity. The first of the WHO targets for the European region was that: 'By the year 2000, the actual differences in health status between countries and between groups within countries should be reduced by at least 25%, by improving the levels of health of disadvantaged nations and groups' (quoted by Radical Statistics Health Group 1991, p. 14).

In many countries strategies for achieving targets for health have included equity as a main criterion for selecting priorities, but not so in Britain (except to the extent that the first *Health of the Nation* criterion states that the areas chosen should be a major problem either in the population as a whole or 'amongst specific groups of people'). The failure to include equity as a separate target in the *Health of the Nation* has been criticized in many quarters (Akehurst et al 1991, Radical Statistics Health Group 1991, Royal College of Nursing 1991b). The Royal College of Nursing (1991b, p. 9) has pointed out that:

> There is clear research evidence which shows inequalities in health still exist. This is true in terms of access to the health service, use of health services and outcome of treatment. Targets must take into account the evidence that some types of preventable disease occur more frequently in some groups in society. Reducing the total incidence of a disease in the nation may be welcome but attempts should also be made to reduce the health differentials between groups.

Both the Royal College of Nursing (1991b) and the Radical Statistics Health Group (1991) point out that the absence of equity as a criterion, and the consequent failure to collect data to monitor it, means that the needs of people whose circumstances make it difficult for them to respond to health promotion and health care initiatives may be neglected in favour of the more advantaged in society. There is the real danger that in trying to achieve the *Health of the Nation* targets health promotion efforts will be directed at the more advantaged sections of society where it is known that such efforts are more likely to pay off; and other health care initiatives too may fail to reach the most disadvantaged in society. The failure to monitor inequalities in health means that any overall reduction in, for example, rates of heart disease, may well mask widening differentials between different social groups.

The criterion of equity has many dimensions. There are issues surrounding not only equity between affluent and deprived sections of society, but also, for example, between the young and the old. Had equity between different age groups been an objective, then the care and rehabilitation of the elderly, and the care of children, may have gained greater prominence (Akehurst et al 1991; Royal College of Nursing 1991a). There is also the question of equity between different client groups. For example, the RCN has pointed to the neglect of people with learning difficulties in the final *Health of the Nation* targets (Royal College of Nursing 1991b).

Equity between those living in different geographical areas is a further issue that the *Health of the Nation* fails to confront. Akehurst et al suggest that it may be appropriate to re-direct resources to combat, for example, heart disease and lung cancer away from District Health Authorities where rates are relatively low, towards Districts with particularly high rates of these illnesses. No such geographical re-distribution of resources is considered in the *Health of the Nation* because equity between different geographical areas, which might entail different targets for different areas, was not an objective (Akehurst et al 1991). Finally, there is nothing in the *Health of the Nation* about equity between different ethnic groups.

## Recent approaches to inequity by central government

It is unclear why originally the *Health of the Nation* chose not to pursue the objective of equity. The Green Paper states only that the reasons for inequalities in health are complex and that there exist no panaceas (Department of Health 1991a). The Green Paper, while recognizing that inequalities in health are widespread, devolves the task of redressing them down to District Health Authorities without any convincing explanation why this issue should be tackled only locally and not at the national level (Department of Health 1991a). However, two publications at the end of 1995 suggest that government has taken seriously the many criticisms of its *Health of the Nation* strategy in terms of the absence of any reference to issues of equity. *On the State of the Public Health 1994* (Department of Health 1995b) observes:

> Significant variations in health may be observed in relation to geographical area, ethnicity, social class, occupation and gender. Such variations, which occur within England and internationally, present a challenge when their underlying causes can be identified and indicate potential for improvement. However, even when the reasons for such variations are known, it may be difficult to achieve improvement through health care interventions alone (Department of Health 1995b, pp. 64–65).

*On the State of the Public Health 1994* goes on to note the launch of a new centre for Health and Society, at University College London Medical School during 1994, at which papers were presented on health variations and their possible causes, and the potential of research on the socio-economic approach to prevention.

The apparent re-naming of 'inequities, or inequalities, in health' by the term *variations in health* is reinforced by the Department of Health's further 1995 publication of a report of that name. *Variations in Health: What can the Department of Health and the NHS do?* (Department of Health 1995c) presents data in support of the observations made in the *Report of the Chief Medical Officer 1994* on substantial variations in health (or rather illness) experienced by geographical location, age, gender, social class and ethnicity. In its executive summary, *Variations in Health* reinforces the following points:

(i) the importance of the purchasing function in identifying population groups who suffer the worst health, and in targeting resources where needs are greatest;

(ii) the need to provide responsive and accessible services to all population groups. This includes identifying, and overcoming, barriers to accessing services on the part of some groups; reducing avoidable variations in treatment outcome by the speedy adoption of best clinical practice; and providing special services and treatment to meet the special needs faced by some groups;

(iii) that it is key that interventions should be effective. To improve knowledge about effectiveness, NHS purchasers should evaluate the impact of interventions intended to reduce variations in health, with particular reference to cost-effectiveness;

(iv) the need to work in alliance with other bodies, including local authorities, the voluntary sector, and communities and individuals themselves. This is especially important given the many and complex factors which contribute to variations in health. (Department of Health 1995c: Executive summary)

Thus it appears that, in future, the government's evaluation of the *Health of the Nation* strategy will incorporate matters concerning variations in health.

## THE TARGETS

The *Health of the Nation* stresses that targets must be measurable, so that it is possible to see the extent to which they are being achieved.

There are however problems with targets. Smith has summarized these problems. First, targets may lead to spurious priority being given to that which is measurable. Second, they may represent an over-simple description of policy. Third, they may appear unrealistic and be easily dismissed as unattainable (Smith 1991a).

The *Health of the Nation* does itself appear to recognize some of these problems. In relation to the attainability of targets the Green Paper states: 'a target which is beyond realistic expectations may...be a disincentive to action' (Department of Health 1991a, p. 33, para 5.22), and '(Targets) must be sufficiently challenging, yet not so daunting that they become a disincentive to achievement' (Department of Health 1991a, p. v).

On the question of giving priority to that which is measurable, the Green Paper states (Department of Health 1991a, p. 33, para 5.23):

'...An indicator for an improvement in coronary heart disease might be a decline in the death rate from that disease. In many cases appropriate indicators of progress are much less obvious – the sort of things which may easily be measured may not be measures of genuine success'.

However, although the *Health of the Nation* shows an awareness of the pitfalls of targets it does not in any way avoid these pitfalls.

## Quantitative versus qualitative targets: a 'spurious emphasis on the measurable'?

It is undoubtedly the case that the *Health of the Nation* targets are narrowly confined to those things which are easily measured. Of the total of 25 separate targets (comprising the 15 'main' targets and the 10 'risk factor' targets – see Boxes 4.1 and 4.2, pp 54–55), all bar a single one (the first mental health target) are quantitative measures of either death rates, the prevalence of illnesses/problems, or the proportion of people engaging in 'unhealthy' behaviours.

The *Health of the Nation* claims to be concerned with both quantity and quality. Its own stated aim of improving the health of the nation is said to involve not only adding 'years to life' but also adding 'life to years' (Department of Health 1992). However, the targets which were eventually chosen are overwhelmingly concerned only with the former aim of prolonging life. The RCN has been critical of this failure to include targets which are directed towards less tangible, more qualitative health gains (Royal College of Nursing 1991a). The RCN has suggested a number of 'quality of life' targets. For example, alongside the

*Health of the Nation* cancer targets, which are exclusively about reducing premature illness and death, targets could have been set which were related to pain control and the delivery of care at a patient's home (Royal College of Nursing 1991b). Such targets may do nothing to reduce the incidence of cancer, but they are important in enhancing the quality of terminally ill patients' lives. The RCN has stressed that much nursing care, for example with elderly people and people with learning disabilities (who are nowhere reflected in the *Health of the Nation* targets) is not about prolonging life but is rather about enhancing quality of life (Royal College of Nursing 1991b). Concern must remain, therefore, that current government policy on health needs assessment is overly concerned with 'cure' to the neglect of 'care'.

## Individual behaviour and the social causes of ill-health

The *Health of the Nation* has been much criticized for failing to address the social and political circumstances which result in much ill-health, and for over-emphasizing the importance of individual behaviour. The Secretary of State for Health, William Waldegrave, in his foreword to the 1991 Green Paper, makes no apology for the emphasis on individual behaviour (Department of Health 1991a, pp. iv–v): '...there is considerable emphasis in this document on the need for people to change their behaviour – whether on smoking, alcohol consumption, exercise, diet, avoidance of accidents and, with AIDS, sexual behaviour. The reason is simple. We live in an age where many of these main causes of premature death and unnecessary disease are related to how we live our lives'.

However, critics argue that the strategy over-emphasizes individual responsibility without sufficiently considering the barriers which make it difficult for some people to change their lifestyle. Critics point out that many illnesses and health-damaging behaviours are related to socio-economic factors of which the *Health of the Nation* takes no account (Radical Statistics Health Group 1991, Akehurst et al 1991). There are limits to what the individual can do in the face of unemployment, poverty and other health hazards, such as the hazards associated with road traffic (Royal College of Nursing 1991b).

## The targets: an 'over-simple description of policy'?

### Individual responsibility versus government action

The Secretary for State, William Waldegrave, in his foreword to the

1991 Green Paper, continues (Department of Health 1991a, pp. iv–v): 'For too long…the health debate has been bedevilled by the two extreme claims of, on the one hand "It's all up to individuals" and, on the other "It's all up to Government". We need a proper balance between individual responsibility and Government action.'

Critics argue that the balance of responsibility for achieving the *Health of the Nation* targets is weighted too heavily towards the individual, with government failing to acknowledge some of its responsibility. The Radical Statistics Health Group, the RCN and Akehurst et al all suggest that individual responsibility for health could be greatly strengthened by legislation, particularly in relation to smoking and alcohol-related diseases, and in relation to accidents. The *Health of the Nation* contains no proposals to introduce tax regimes which discourage smoking and alcohol consumption; no proposals to introduce legislation to control tobacco advertising; no proposals to introduce random breath testing; and no proposals to introduce and enforce measures related to road safety (Radical Statistics Health Group 1991, Royal College of Nursing 1991a,b, Smith 1991a).

## The Health of the Nation: a 'concerted effort'?

The *Health of the Nation* stresses throughout that 'health' is not simply the product of the health services but is the responsibility on an array of individuals and organizations. However, there has been much criticism of the strategy for failing to follow through its own belief in concerted action. The 1991 Green Paper acknowledges that in the past, it has been concerted action on a range of fronts which has brought about improvements in the nations' health. In relation to the dramatic reduction in infectious diseases which was accomplished in the late 19th and early 20th centuries, the Green Paper states that (Department of Health 1991a, p. 1): '…the achievement was essentially due to various social and public health changes. Safe water and sewerage, better housing, less overcrowding and better working conditions, greater economic prosperity, more effective methods of family planning, better nutrition and better education lay at the heart of the transformation'.

Yet nowhere in the *Health of the Nation* are the kinds of policies which brought about such dramatic health gains in the past advocated for today. The Radical Statistics Health Group argues that the kinds of health promotion activities pursued solely within the NHS advocated in the *Health of the Nation* are unlikely to improve the nation's health. They believe that (Radical Statistics Health Group 1991, p. 12): 'Concerted action is needed from many government departments with policies to reduce homelessness, increase income support, protect the environment including reduction of air and water pollution, improve public transport, and promote health and safety at work . . . '.

Thus, the *Health of the Nation*, while describing a century of achievements related to public health measures, better housing and greater economic prosperity, contains none of the kinds of policies required to combat the adverse effect on health of growing poverty, homelessness and unemployment (Radical Statistics Health Group 1991).

## Measures of the nation's health

The RCN has questioned the use of narrow medical data, such as mortality rates, as the best 'measuring-stick' fo the nation's health. They have advocated instead the use of deprivation indices, such as unemployment rates, which are strongly associated with poor health (Royal College of Nursing 1991a; see also Ch. 3). In advocating the use of deprivation measures instead of mortality rates, the RCN is underlining their belief that major improvements in health result not simply from exhortations to individuals to change their life-styles but also from policies directed at the social causes of ill-health.

## Health and disease

A final criticism of the *Health of the Nation* targets is that they are about disease rather than health, with the emphasis on narrow medical targets (Radical Statistics Health Group 1991, pp. 10–12; Royal College of Nursing 1991a, p. 1). The *Health of the Nation* appears implicitly to rely on a definition of health as the absence of disease, rather than a more positive definition of health (Royal College of Nursing 1991b, p. 3): 'By focusing on disease levels and treatment options as goals, the health of the nation gives a message that more treatment is needed rather than more health.'

Even the mental health target is restricted to a narrow concern with the 'social functioning' of mentally ill people rather than expressing a wider concern with empowering those with mental health problems to lead more socially fulfilling lives (see also Radical Statistics Health Group's discussion of the Green Paper's definition of disability 1991).

## Unrealistic targets?

Cynics have suggested that targets are, at worst, a means of diverting political attention away from the difficulties of the NHS and at best are no more than empty sloganizing (Smith 1991a, Mooney 1994). Although a number of commentators are critical of the failure to provide more resources to achieve targets, it is acknowledged even among its critics that target-setting is useful in focusing attention on what needs to be done and how to go about doing it. None of the specific *Health of the Nation* targets has been subject to the charge that it is unrealistic and unattainable. On the contrary, it has been suggested that the targets might foster complacency. Akehurst et al point out that when performance indicators were introduced into the NHS they did not encourage those Districts and Units which were performing well to improve. One danger in the *Health of the Nation* targets, Akehurst et al suggest, is that agencies will engage in activities where targets can be met easily, rather than those where the most real gains are to be made (Akehurst et al 1991).

## THE *HEALTH OF THE NATION*: CONCLUSION

The *Health of the Nation* contains both strengths and weaknesses. From the perspective of economists, its greatest weakness is its failure to weigh up the costs and benefits of different interventions, and thus its failure to provide a 'rational' basis for determining priorities in the allocation of health care resources. From the perspectives of both epidemiology and sociology its greatest weaknesses is its failure to address inequalities in health and inequities in the way in which resources are distributed between different sections in society. From the perspective of nurses, its major weakness is its concentration on the goal of increasing longevity to the neglect of the goal of enhancing the quality of life.

However, the strategy has many strengths. First, it recognizes the importance of preventive, and not only curative, interventions in improving health. Second, it recognizes that health is the responsibility not only of the formal health care services but of a wide range of individuals and organizations. Finally, it is a strength of the *Health of the Nation* that it adopts a target-setting approach. Targets make visible what might otherwise remain obscured, they provide a basis for shared goals and shared values, they give direction to what might otherwise be un-coordinated action, and they provide a basis for monitoring and evaluating the effects of interventions designed to improve health.

## HEALTH NEEDS ASSESSMENT: GOVERNMENT GUIDANCE TO DISTRICT HEALTH AUTHORITIES

In the remainder of this chapter we look at government guidance to local District Health Authorities for assessing the needs of the local populations they serve. The *Health of the Nation* Green Paper (Department of Health 1991a) stresses that District Health Authorities have an important role to play in bringing about improvements in health. The Green Paper states that the responsibilities of District Health Authorities, as 'champions of the people' are three-fold (Department of Health 1991a, p. iii): 'First, to assess the state of health of the people they serve. Second, to obtain the services needed to ensure effective action is taken to maintain good health, prevent and treat ill-health, rehabilitate people to good health, and provide support and care for those who are disabled, chronically ill or dying. Third, to ensure the quality and effectiveness – including cost effectiveness – of the services their residents use'.

Much of the government's guidance to District Health Authorities has been issued through the National Health Service Executive (NHSE, formerly known as the National Health Service Management Executive (NHSME)). Below, we look in some detail at the NHSME's recommendations to local District Health Authorities for assessing health needs.

### Introduction

#### *The NHS reforms: purchasers and providers*
Two recent government policy documents have shaped the way in which the needs for health and social care will be assessed in the future in the United Kingdom: *Caring for People* (Department of Health 1989a) and *Working for Patients* (Department of Health 1989b). These two White Papers became law in the 1990 National Health Service (NHS) and Community Care Act.

The NHS reforms introduced in the 1990 Act are structured around one central theme: the separation of the *purchaser* and the *provider* role. Within the NHS the main purchasers of health care services are local District Health Authorities and local Family Health Service Authorities. In this section we look only at the role of District Health Authorities. The role of purchasing District Health Authorities is to assess the health needs of the populations they serve, and to determine the resources to be allocated to various services in order to secure improvements in the population's health. In discharging their role, purchasers set up agreements or contracts with providers, such as hospitals and community units who then deliver the services required (Akehurst & Ferguson 1993; Downie & Calman 1994; Raftery & Stevens 1994).

**Government guidance to District Health Authorities.** In a 1991 discussion paper, the NHSME recommended to District Health Authorities (DHAs) that they should adopt a 'hybrid approach' to health needs assessment (NHSME 1991). This should incorporate both a 'strict approach' which draws on the disciplines of epidemiology and economics, and a 'pragmatic approach' which recognizes that in the 'real world' it is not always possible, or desirable, to remain within a 'strict' approach. Adopting a 'pragmatic approach' means that epidemiological and economic standpoints must be supplemented by the viewpoints of a range of groups and agencies with an interest in health needs assessment. The pragmatic approach also recognizes that most of the appropriate epidemiological and economic information for assessing health needs is often lacking, particularly at the local level at which purchasers operate.

The NHSME envisaged three separate but related elements of health needs assessment. The first element involved undertaking an epidemiological assessment of the population's need for effective and cost-effective health care services. The second and third elements were more pragmatic. The second was to draw comparisons between Districts or between providers in the same District. The third element was to adopt a 'corporate stance' to needs assessment which takes into account the views, demands, wishes and alternative perspectives of interested parties (NHS Management-Executive 1991).

Before looking in more depth at these three elements of health needs assessment, it is helpful to look first at some of the general issues relating to health needs assessment discussed in the National Health Service Management Executive's (NHSME's) (1991) discussion paper.

**The need for health and the need for health care.** The NHSME's (1991) discussion paper defines health care needs as 'the ability to benefit' from health care or preventive services. A distinction is drawn between the need for health and the need for health care. The need for health is a broad concept. Health needs are met not only by health care services but also through other public services and policies, such as housing and environmental policies, as well as through broad environmental and social changes. The need for health care is more specific. Health care needs are met through health care services.

**Need, demand and supply.** Further distinctions are drawn in the NHSME's (1991) discussion paper between 'need', 'demand' and 'supply'. A person might 'demand' antibiotics, but she does not 'need' antibiotics because they are totally ineffective in treating viral infections. In other words, people who do not have the 'ability to benefit' from antibiotics are not in need of them. The supply of health care is different from the need and the demand for health care. The supply of health care is simply what is provided but this does not necessarily correspond with what people need or demand (see also Bradshaw 1972a, Stevens & Gabbay 1991).

**The benefits of health care.** The NHSME (1991) paper acknowledges that whether or not a person is in need of health care – whether or not they have the 'ability to benefit' from health care – depends on what is defined as of benefit. A narrow interpretation would suggest that only those health care interventions which bring about a measurable improvement in people's clinical health status are of benefit. However, such a narrow definition of benefit would exclude many 'caring' aspects of health care which have no impact on a person's clinical health status. It would exclude the provision of comfort or reassurance to patients and health care workers; for example a diagnostic test might reassure a patient and her GP, and even antibiotics might reassure someone with a viral infection, inappropriately, that 'something is being done'. A narrow interpretation of benefit would also exclude the care and support of patients with chronic conditions or terminal illnesses where there is no possibility of altering the natural history of the illness (Culyer 1977). Additionally, it would exclude benefits which might accrue not to patients, but to their relatives. The NHSME does not employ such a narrow definition of health benefits. Their definition includes not only changes in clinical health status, but also reassurance, supportive care to patients and the relief of pressure on their lay carers (NHS Management Executive 1991).

## The three elements of needs assessment

**Epidemiological needs assessment.** The epidemiological approach to needs assessment is said by the NHSME (1991) to rely on knowledge about three things:

- the local level (incidence and prevalence) of various diseases or health problems;
- the effectiveness of interventions to treat these diseases;
- the cost-effectiveness of such interventions.

Thus, what the NHSME describes as an epidemiological approach to needs assessment is in essence a combination of a strict epidemiological approach which looks at the size of the problem and the effectiveness of interventions; and an economic element which looks at cost-effectiveness. The NHSME's approach thus emphasizes the question of how much of a problem there is (incidence and prevalence); and how well it can be dealt with (effectiveness and cost-effectiveness) (NHS Management Executive 1991, Raftery & Stevens 1994). The relative importance of these two aspects – how much of a problem there is, versus the effectiveness of treatments – is said by the NHSME to vary. If there is reason to doubt the effectiveness of an intervention then effectiveness is the more important matter to investigate. If a service is of proven effectiveness then the important question is whether it is reaching all those who need it – whether it is distributed equitably (NHS Management Executive 1991).

Data sources for the epidemiological approach include demographic and social data, such as local mortality and morbidity statistics, and statistics about levels of deprivation, as well as data concerning effectiveness and cost-effectiveness of services.

Many of the data for an epidemiological approach to needs assessment are either lacking or deficient. For example, mortality and morbidity statistics are often deficient for the purpose of relating the burden of health problems to health care services. This is because changes in mortality and morbidity rates reflect not only changes in health care interventions but also changes in broad public policy and other environmental and social change. Hence mortality data allow us to monitor whether the population is becoming more healthy, but a healthier population is not the result solely of the provision of health-care services. Data about the effectiveness of services are often simply absent. Local purchasers must instead rely on measures of supply and demand, such as service–utilization rates, or waiting lists. These are proxy measures for effectiveness. The assumption is that if there is a great demand for services (as measured through waiting lists) or if the service is heavily used (as measured through service–utilization rates), then these services must be effective. Of course such an assumption cannot be made and the NHSME recognizes this. Such data are used for pragmatic reasons in the absence of data which give a better indication of whether or not services are effective. Finally, there exist very few studies of cost-effectiveness. Local purchasers must often rely simply on information about costs in the absence of information which relates costs to outcomes.

**Comparative assessment.** Epidemiological assessment involves comparing the burden of illness with the ability to deal with it effectively and cost-effectively. Comparative assessment involves comparisons either between or within Districts. Comparative assessment relies on Bradshaw's concept of 'comparative need' (see Ch. 2). If people with the same characteristics in different Districts are not receiving the same services, those who are not receiving the service can be viewed as in need. Similarly, if one provider within a District is achieving better outcomes than another, those served by the latter provider are in need. The comparative approach advocated by the NHSME relies on the same kind of data which are used in the epidemiological approach, such as mortality and morbidity data, service–utilization rates, waiting times, and, where they exist, data about effectiveness.

**The corporate approach.** Competing views on needs cannot be dismissed, and local District Health Authorities are expected by the NHSME (1991) to make 'healthy alliances' with other informed agencies and individuals, including GPs, other providers, health care workers and local people; as well as Regional Health Authorities and the NHSME itself (NHS Management Executive 1991, Raftery & Stevens 1994). Thus a 'strict approach' to health needs assessment which relies on epidemiology and economics must be complemented by a 'pragmatic approach' which takes into account the views and opinions of other interested parties. Subsequent guidance from the NHSME (NHS Management Executive 1992) on gathering and using the views of local people suggests that it is important to listen to local people, discuss their views, keep them informed and report back to them.

## Discussion of the NHSME's approach to health needs assessment

### The benefits of health care

The NHSME acknowledges that there are many benefits of health care besides improved clinical health status. What is defined as a benefit is crucial to nurses because their work involves many caring interventions the benefits of which relate to the process of health care delivery rather than to clinical outcomes. The importance of including more than a change in clinical health status as a measure of benefit is underlined when it is realized that in developed countries people place their greatest demands on health-care services during the last few months of their lives and yet care for irreversible illness contributes almost nothing to life expectancy (Drummond 1993). Thus, health care services are not only about increasing life-expectancy, they are also about providing for a 'dignified death'. Moreover the 'need' for health care is a holistic need, not only for physical care but also for psychological and spiritual sustenance.

Although the NHSME recognizes the diversity of potential benefits of health care, in practice benefits do tend to be defined in a narrow way, and in terms of quantifiable outcomes rather than more intangible processes. This is partly because, in investigating the effectiveness of different health care interventions, people tend to measure only those things which are easily measurable. It is a *relatively* simple matter to examine the effectiveness of a drug by comparing the physiological outcome of taking the drug with the outcome of not taking the drug. It is another matter to measure the ability to benefit from the psychological and spiritual care given to a terminally-ill patient.

It should by now be clear that the concept of benefit or health gain is not value-neutral. What counts as a benefit is open to wide interpretation, involving value-judgements about what kinds of outcomes we value and aspire to achieve. The NHSME's approach does recognize the diversity of potential benefits of health care, but, in reality, as we have seen above in our discussion of the *Health of the Nation*, the benefits which are pursued by governments and local purchasers tend to be those with the most measurable outcomes.

### Need, demand and the 'corporate approach'

The NHSME's discussion document (1991) distinguishes between 'demand' and 'need'. Here, we would wish to stress that resolving conflicts between the two is not a straightforward matter. In Chapter 2 we noted Bradshaw's distinction between 'expressed need' (what people demand) and 'normative need' (what the expert or professional defines as need). Similarly, in our discussion of economic concepts in Chapter 2, we saw that 'demand' expresses the idea that the consumer is sovereign, whereas 'need' expresses the idea that consumers cannot always be sovereign because they lack information, so that elite bodies such as the health care professions are sometimes in a better position to decide what their 'needs' are (Mooney 1992). Thus the distinction between 'need' and 'demand' raises questions about *who decides* what counts as a need and what is a demand (Akehurst & Ferguson 1993, Mooney 1994, Downie & Calman 1994). In the NHSME's own example we might come down on the side of the expert and agree that people with viral infections do not need antibiotics. However, there are other instances where patients or nurses might feel that a patient has a need for a particular service, but the patient's doctor, or the local District Health Authority, or even the government, feels the patient is demanding a service which she does not need (or which cannot be afforded). For example, patients with psychological disorders may feel they have a need for counselling or psychotherapy, but doctors or the local District Health Authority might feel that patients do not have the ability to benefit from counselling or psychotherapy for which there is only scant and contradictory evidence of their effectiveness. A doctor might feel that the patient has a need for drug therapy but counselling is simply a demand and not a 'real' need. We cannot get away from the fact that the distinction between a demand and a need is a value judgement over which outright conflicts do arise.

Adopting the 'corporate stance' is the NHSME's way of accommodating competing viewpoints. However, there are dangers in the adoption of a corporate stance. Cynics might argue that the NHSME's model amounts to nothing more than a cosmetic exercise with no adequate mechanism for integrating the consumer voice with other aspects of the Dictrict Health Authority's role (see Akehurst & Ferguson 1993). As we have suggested already, there may be a mismatch between perceptions of need on the part of policy makers, professionals and lay people. It is not clear how conflicts between these different perceptions can be resolved when resources are finite and not all the needs identified by local people themselves can be met (Pollock 1992). There is no solution to this problem. Meeting all the needs identified by local people themselves invariably gives rise to the 'bottomless pit' problem (Chadwick 1994). Although it is clearly important to take account of the views expressed by local people, it is equally clear that not all of their needs or demands can be met. A second difficulty with the 'corporate approach' is that it may encourage those consumers most able to register their demands or needs to do so at the expense of those less able to articulate their needs (Percy-Smith & Sanderson 1992). A third danger in the NHSME's model is that local purchasing authorities will be influenced not so much by providers, health workers and local people, but rather by the NHSME, since the NHSME includes itself in its 1991 discussion document as an interested party whose views must be taken into account (NHS Management Executive 1991). Thus, what the NHSME document blandly describes as adopting a 'pragmatic' approach means, in effect, that District Health Authorities must take into account the concerns and political priorities of central government, as expressed through the NHSME via such initiatives as the Patients' Charter (NHS Management Executive 1991). This is an aspect of the NHSME's approach to which a number of economists take exception. Akehurst & Ferguson (1993) suggest that taking into account the views of central government may commit local District Health Authorities to meeting trivial health needs at the expense of more important needs. Economists point to the way in which bodies such as the NHSME impose political constraints on purchasing authorities, in the form, for example, of waiting list initiatives. Such initiatives may commit District Health Authorities to reducing waiting lists for relatively minor conditions such as varicose veins, while neglecting to reduce the waiting lists for, for example, hip replacement surgery, in an effort to bring about an overall reduction in waiting times. In advocating a 'corporate approach' the NHSME is attempting to ensure that health needs assessment is not based on the covert assumptions of particular academic disciplines, such as economics, but rather that it is based on the value-judgements and political priorities of a wider cross-section of society (see Richardson 1994). However, we have seen that some economists' view is that policy is in danger of being unduly influenced by the political priorities of government. While we ourselves do not subscribe to a conspiracy theory that government is subverting the process of health needs assessment, it is nevertheless important to recognize that there is no simple recipe for resolving differences between competing interest and viewpoints. What is important is continuing debate between all parties and disciplines to ensure that no one vested interest carries undue influence.

## CONCLUSION

The NHSME is right to stress that health needs assessment is not a technical problem for which either economics or epidemiology has all the answers. Information on which to base both epidemiological and economic approaches to health needs assessment is lacking, and neither discipline can provide a formula for assessing health needs. We have seen that as a means of accommodating competing approaches the government recommends a 'hybrid' approach which draws on the disciplines of economics and epidemiology but also takes 'pragmatic' account of the concerns of all those parties with an interest in health needs assessment. However, there is no simple way of reconciling competing perceptions of need.

In the following three chapters we explore further some of the issues raised in this chapter. In Chapter 5 we examine the basis for the criticism of the *Health of the Nation* that it fails to address inequalities in health. Chapter 5 looks at the argument that policy should be concerned not only with reducing the burden of ill-health in the population but also with redressing inequalities in health. In Chapters 6 and 7 we look in greater depth at the two disciplines of epidemiology and economics, on which health needs assessment relies.

# Inequalities in health and health care

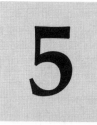

5

## CONTENTS

## INTRODUCTION

We saw in the previous chapter that the aim of the *Health of the Nation* was to reduce the total burden of ill-health in the nation. However, many people argue that if the burden of ill-health is to be reduced then policy must address questions concerning the relationship between ill-health and its wider social causes such as poverty, low income and unemployment (see Black 1994, Bradshaw 1994). It is argued that only if we understand the relationship between health and its social causes can we begin to develop appropriate strategies to improve the population's health and to reduce inequalities between different groups in society.

In this chapter we explore the sociological approach to health needs assessment. The emphasis in the sociological approach is on the wider, social determinants of health, and on documenting inequalities which exist in both the distribution of health problems and the use of health care services. The sociological approach is central to health needs assessment because of its concern to bring about greater equality in health, and a more equitable distribution of health-care resources.

This chapter looks at the evidence that there exist inequalities in health between different groups in society, and considers the various arguments which have been put forward to explain these inequalities. The chapter explores the policy implications of different explanations for inequalities in health, and concludes by discussing what should be done (if anything) in policy terms to reduce inequalities in health.

## INEQUALITIES IN HEALTH

The publication of the *Black Report* in 1980 and *The Health Divide* in 1987 represent important landmarks in our knowledge and understanding of inequalities in health. (These two reports are reproduced in Townsend & Davidson (1992).) In the following sections we document the main findings of these two reports, and of subsequent research into inequalities in health.

### Geographical inequalities

Both the *Black Report* and *The Health Divide* have drawn attention to differences in death rates between different geographical areas in the UK, and to the North/South gradient in health experiences (Townsend & Davidson 1992).

In attempting to explain geographical inequalities in health, the

**Table 5.1** Mortality of men and women in different regions of Britain (1979–80 plus 1982–3)

| | Direct age-standardized death rate 1000 | | |
| Region | Men (20–64) | Single women (20–59) | Married women (20–59) |
|---|---|---|---|
| Central Clydeside | 7.86 | 1.78 | 3.23 |
| Strathclyde | 7.14 | 1.66 | 3.06 |
| North | 6.43 | 1.56 | 2.50 |
| North-West | 6.37 | 1.69 | 2.52 |
| Remainder of Scotland | 6.13 | 1.47 | 2.58 |
| Wales | 5.86 | 1.43 | 2.34 |
| Yorkshire and Humberside | 5.83 | 1.48 | 2.32 |
| West Midlands | 5.72 | 1.54 | 2.26 |
| East Midlands | 5.28 | 1.40 | 2.14 |
| South-East | 4.88 | 1.29 | 1.97 |
| South-West | 4.82 | 1.32 | 1.93 |
| East Anglia | 4.37 | 1.14 | 1.79 |
| Scotland | 6.92 | 1.62 | 2.89 |
| England and Wales | 5.43 | 1.41 | 2.17 |
| Britain | 5.57 | 1.43 | 2.23 |

Source: Townsend & Davidson (1992, p 246). Reproduced with permission from Whitehead M 1987 The Health Divide. HMSO, London.

*Black Report* viewed social class, or socio-economic status as a key concept. Geographical variations reflect, to an extent, differences in social class or socio-economic status between different regions of the country. Notwithstanding the mix of social classes within each region, in general, it is in Scotland and the North of England where those in the lower social classes are concentrated. Hence geographical differences between regions can be explained partly as a reflection of social class differences (Whitehead (1987) in Townsend & Davidson (1992)).

## Socio-economic inequalities and health

The *Black Report* found there to be a marked gradient in health experience between social classes. Figure 5.1 shows that, for all major causes of death, mortality is greater in class V than in class 1.

Significant differences in death rates between different socio-economic classes have been shown to exist in many studies since the publication of the *Black Report*. In a review of research conducted since the *Black Report*, a recent King's Fund report quotes the following selection of findings (Benzeval et al 1995, p. 4):

- The total excess deaths in the most disadvantaged half of the population is equivalent to a major aircrash or shipwreck every day (Jacobson et al 1991).

- There would be 42 000 fewer deaths each year for people aged 15–74 if the death rate of people with manual jobs was the same as for those in non-manual occupations (Jacobson et al 1991).

- A child from an unskilled social class is twice as likely to die before the age of 15 as a child with a professional father (Woodroffe et al 1993).

- If the whole population had experienced the same death rate as the non-manual classes, there would have been 700 fewer stillbirths and 1500 fewer deaths in the first year of life in England and Wales in 1988 (Delamothe 1991).

### Trends in inequalities in health over time

The *Black Report* found not only that there existed inequalities between social classes but also that some of these inequalities widened over time. The *Black Report* observed that 'Between 1949/53 and 1959/63 inequalities between the highest- and lowest-ranking occupational classes in mortality experience appear to have widened' (the *Black Report*, in Townsend & Davidson 1992).

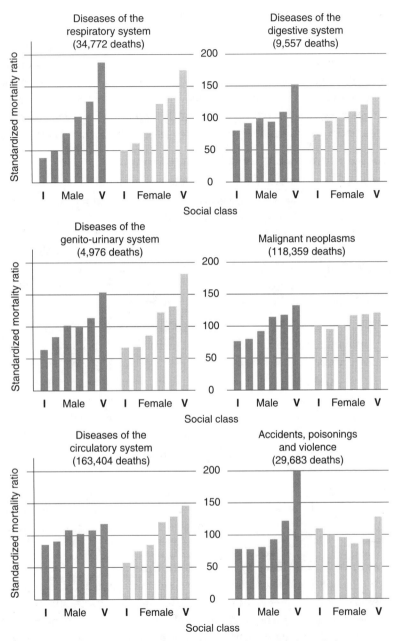

**Fig. 5.1** Occupational class and mortality in adult life (men and married women 15–64) by husband's occupation. Source: Townsend & Davidson (1992, p 47). Reproduced with permission from Black D Sir 1980 The Black Report. HMSO, London.

**Table 5.2** Mortality of men by occupational class (1930s–1970s) (standardized mortality ratios)

| Occupational class | | | Men aged 15–64 | | | |
|---|---|---|---|---|---|---|
| | | | 1959–63 unadjusted | | 1970–72 unadjusted | |
| | 1930–32 | 1949–53* | | adjusted† | | adjusted |
| I Professional | 90 | 86 | 76 | 75 | 77 | 75 |
| II Managerial | 94 | 92 | 81 | — | 81 | — |
| III Skilled manual and non-manual | 97 | 101 | 100 | — | 104 | — |
| IV Partly skilled | 102 | 104 | 103 | — | 114 | — |
| V Unskilled | 111 | 118 | 143 | 127 | 137 | 121 |

*Corrected figures as published in *Registrar General's Decennial Supplement England and Wales, 1961: Occupational Mortality Tables*, London, HMSO, 1971, p. 22.
†Occupations in 1959–63 and 1970–72 have been reclassified according to the 1950 classification.
Source: Townsend & Davidson (1992, p 59). Reproduced with permission from Black D Sir 1980 The Black Report. HMSO, London.

Much of the furore which followed the original publication of the *Black Report* in 1980 centred around this finding of widening differentials between occupational classes. Later in this chapter we discuss the criticisms which this finding has provoked.

## Deprivation and health

The concepts of social class, socio-economic status, and deprivation have all been used at various times to explain inequalities in health. All three concepts are attempts to encapsulate those social, economic and material circumstances which are associated with poor health. In documenting inequalities in health the *Black Report* relied very largely on the concept of social class, using 'occupational class' as an indicator of social class. However, since the publication of the *Black Report* there has been a proliferation of studies which have relied on indicators of deprivation, such as unemployment or low income, rather than occupation to measure inequalities in health (see Ch. 3). These studies confirm that whatever measure is chosen, a similar pattern emerges, with those in the less well-off sections of society faring worse than their better-off contemporaries. In particular, research undertaken by Townsend, Phillimore and Beattie (Townsend et al 1988, Phillimore et al 1994), which relied on indicators other than occupational class, has shown, in the North of England, a similar pattern of inequalities to that shown in the *Black Report*. Moreover, like the *Black Report*, this study provided evidence of widening inequalities. The widening of inequalities documented by Black during the 1950s was also evident in the 1980s.

## CASE STUDY I

*Widening Inequality of Health in Northern England, 1981–91*, Phillimore et al (1994)

### Summary of findings
The study found that in electoral wards in the Northern region, inequalities in mortality had widened in men and women in all age groups under 75 years between 1981 and 1991. This was mainly because the situation in the poorest areas was worsening relative to the rest of the population. In absolute terms, mortality fell in the most affluent areas, while in some age categories in the poorest areas it increased, especially in men aged 15–44.

### Project design
Census data for 1981 and 1991 was used to rank 678 wards in the North of England on an index of material deprivation. The index was made up of four variables: unemployment, car ownership, housing tenure and household over-crowding. Standardized mortality ratios were calculated for various periods between 1981 and 1991, and for different age categories.

### Discussion of findings
The most striking finding was the evidence of the poorest areas increasingly coming adrift from the experience of the rest of the population. In the poorest one-fifth of electoral wards included in the study, mortality had worsened in relative terms. However, even excluding the experience of the most deprived fifth of electoral wards, there had been no narrowing of inequality in mortality across the remainder of the population.

## Indicators of health

It will have been noted that most of the health inequalities discussed in the *Black Report* and *The Health Divide*, and in many subsequent studies, are inequalities in death rates – the extreme of the health continuum. Undoubtedly one of the reasons for this pre-occupation with the negative aspects of health is the fact that mortality rates are both available and unequivocal (see Ch. 3). However, both the *Black Report* and *The Health Divide* found inequalities in illness or morbidity, and such findings have been repeated in subsequent studies. For example,

Breeze et al (1991) found evidence of a socio-economic gradient in most of the causes of chronic illness and disability, with the highest rates among those in manual occupations (Benzeval et al 1995). A number of national surveys have demonstrated socio-economic differences in morbidity and risk factors (Gregory et al 1990, Power et al 1991, Benzeval et al 1994).

The *Black Report* was aware of the limitations of relying solely on mortality and morbidity rates which measure only negative health, and called for the development and use of measures of positive health. *The Health Divide* reviewed some of the research which had been initiated in this area following the *Black Report* (Townsend & Davidson 1992, pp. 313–315) and there has since been a greater emphasis on measuring aspects of positive health (see Ch. 3).

## Inequalities in access to health services

The *Black Report* drew attention to inequalities not only in health outcomes, as expressed in mortality and morbidity rates, but also to inequalities in access to high-quality health care between different social classes. For every kind of health care, including hospital services, preventive services and primary care services, the *Black Report* showed that there is a class gradient, with those in the higher classes enjoying better access, and better care, than those in the lower classes. The *Black Report's* findings confirmed the earlier, more anecdotal, observation of Tudor Hart, a GP working in a deprived area of Wales, who suggested that those who needed the most care received the least. Tudor Hart termed his observation the 'inverse care law' (Hart 1971):

> In areas with most sickness and death, general practitioners have more work, larger lists, (and) less hospital support . . . ; and hospital doctors shoulder heavier care-loads with less staff and equipment, more obsolete buildings and suffer recurrent crises in the availability of beds and replacement staff. These trends can be summed up as the inverse care law: that the availability of good medical care tends to vary inversely with the need of the population served.

## EXPLANATIONS FOR INEQUALITIES IN HEALTH AND THEIR POLICY IMPLICATIONS

No-one denies that there are marked inequalities in health between different socio-economic groups. However, there is a great deal of debate about the interpretation and explanation of such findings. For example, Klein (1991) is critical of the assumption that simply because a correlation can be documented between membership of occupational class V and poor health, this is evidence that socio-economic deprivation is the cause of poor health. He points out that the higher rates of smoking, or the unhealthy diets consumed by people in social class V could equally well explain this finding.

In this section we examine five types of explanation for the *Black Report's* findings. These are summarized in Table 5.3, which is modified from the explanations given in Chapter 6 of the *Black Report, Towards an Explanation of Health Inequalities* (Townsend & Davidson 1992) and Chapter 6 of *The Health Divide, Explaining Health Inequalities* (Townsend & Davidson 1992). The different explanations do not preclude one another, and they are not exhaustive of all possible explanations. It is important for the purpose of understanding the different explanations, as well as their associated policy implications, to treat each as if it were separate. However, no-one denies that, in the 'real' world, it is not always possible, or helpful, to opt for one type of explanation rather than another. Health workers may frequently find that they are working with two or more types of explanation simultaneously, and this is usually the most productive approach to adequately explaining the often complex situations which they frequently encounter.

In distinguishing between different explanations, both the *Black Report* and *The Health Divide* combine theories of natural selection with those of social selection. In Table 5.3 we differentiate between two types of selection theory: theories of selective social mobility, and theories of natural selection.

### The artefact explanation

Proponents of artefactual explanations argue that research findings do not reflect a real phenomenon, they are just the product of the research instruments and methods used. Hence an explanation in terms of artefact of the *Black Report's* finding of a relationship between occupational class and health would be that 'occupational class' is just an artificially constructed variable, and although there is a correlation or association between occupational class and health, this association is not causal; it is not even meaningful. Of course no-one denies that there are marked inequalities in health between different sections of

**Table 5.3** Explanations for inequalities in health

| Explanation | Theoretical base | Policies required |
|---|---|---|
| 1. Artefact | 'Class' is an artefact of research design | None |
| 2. Material/structural | 'Health' is a dependent variable; 'class', 'poverty' and 'environment' are independent | Political: income maintenance, public health measures |
| 3. Social/cultural | 'Health' is a dependent variable; reckless behaviours (e.g. smoking) are independent | Psychosocial: re-education |
| 4. Selective social mobility | 'Health' is an independent variable, 'class' and 'poverty' are dependent | Biomedical and political: medical intervention and income maintenance |
| 5. Natural selection | 'Inherited predisposition' is an independent variable; 'health' and 'class' are dependent | Bio-medical: screening |

Adapted from the *Black Report*, Chapter 6, and *The Health Divide*, Chapter 6 (Townsend & Davidson 1992).

society. But proponents of artefactual theories question the use of 'occupational class' as an indicator of any meaningful difference between sections of society.

Artefactual explantions have been applied to the *Black Report's* findings of growing inequalities between occupational classes. It will be recalled that the *Black Report* found that inequalities between occupational classes during the period 1959–63 were even wider than inequalities during the period 1949–53 (see above). An artefactual explanation of this finding is that the *apparent* widening of differentials is just that – it is apparent rather than real; it is the result of the way in which the data has been collected and compared, rather than the reflection of any real changes over time. In essence, it is argued that because occupational classes change over time both in their composition and in their size, comparisons over time are not comparing like with like. Moreover, because comparisons between occupational classes are usually comparisons only of those under the age of 65, this is said to exclude those age groups where the greatest increases in life expectancy have been achieved (Illsley, 1987, Klein 1988). Hence, proponents of the artefact explanation believe that the *Black Report* artificially constructs (or at least greatly exaggerates the extent of) changes over time.

If artefactual explanations are accepted it follows that there are no policy consequences arising from them. Policy which aims to address health inequalities in society must flow from measuring differences in health in other ways, that is, in ways which reflect 'real' instead of artefactual differences. If there has not been any widening of differentials over time, then it is not necessary to look for any 'real' causes of, or solutions to, this problem.

The issue of whether the *Black Report's* findings of growing inequalities were simply an artefact continues to be hotly debated today. As we have seen above, recent research challenges artefactual explanations, showing that whatever indicator of socio-economic disadvantage is chosen, be it 'occupational class' or 'car ownership' there is evidence of widening differentials between social groups (Townsend et al 1988, Phillimore et al 1994).

The *material/structural* explanation has commanded vast quantities of research evidence and continues to derive major support from many researchers. This explanation holds that the material and structural circumstances of people's lives (such as poverty, unemployment, poor housing) are real, independent, causative, influences on which health ultimately depends. The policy implications of the material/structural explanation lie in the assumed need for widespread structural change implemented through intersectoral collaboration, for example, through measures taken to reduce poverty (especially among families with young children), to promote employment, and to improve housing. This explanation was rejected by Patrick Jenkins, the Secretary of State for Social Services at the time when the *Black Report* was first published in 1980, and, as we have seen, it has not gained support in subsequent *Health of the Nation* policies. However, material/structural explanations and policies still command widespread support. For example, Townsend and his research team, in their study of inequalities in the North of England (see above) explain their findings as the result of material and structural changes in society during the last decade. They argue that widening income differentials, a growth in the proportion of the population living on less than half of average income, high levels of unemployment, and changes in the state benefit and tax systems, are showing their effects in a failure to reduce inequalities in the population as a whole and the worsening of the health of the poorest sections of society (Phillimore et al 1994).

*Social and cultural* explanations, like the material/structural explanations, see health as the dependent variable. However its dependency is believed to lie not in the material or structural features in the wider society but in the reckless, health damaging behaviour of individuals such as smoking, drinking, lack of exercise, drug-taking etc. It is often argued that such behaviours are *learned* within families or social groups and therefore policies which flow from this explanation tend to emphasise the re-education of individuals in order to encourage more appropriate health-enhancing behaviour. For example, health education programmes designed in such a way as to encourage people to follow healthier life styles. The policy implications which flow from this theoretical perspective can be 'weak' or 'strong'. Clearly the giving of information in an open and democratic form allows individuals to make informed choices regarding health enhancing behaviours. In its 'strong' form however individuals who persist in pursuing health-damaging behaviour may be denied access to certain social benefits, including health care.

Social and cultural explanations for inequalities in health were widely held to be true in government circles during the mid-1970s, when they were thought to explain why policies based on structural/material explanations had not worked. Sir Keith Joseph, when Secretary of State for Social services in 1972, expressed disquiet at the persistence of poverty and social deprivation despite more than 30 years of a welfare state in Britain. In a speech to the Pre-School Playgroup's Association in 1972, he posed the following question (Joseph 1972): 'Why is it that, in spite of long periods of full employment and relative prosperity and the improvement in community services since the Second World War, deprivation and the problems of maladjustment so conspicuously persist?' He suggested that an explanation might lie in the persistence of a 'cycle of deprivation' which he linked to patterns of parenting, suggesting that deprivation and maladjustment might be transmitted from generation to generation resulting ultimately in physical and mental health problems, as well as social problems (Brown & Madge, 1982, p. 1).

As a result of Sir Keith Joseph's hypothesis, a huge (by today's standards) programme of research was initiated which resulted in 10 years of academic inquiry. Unfortunately, the results were equivocal. Some individuals were born into deprived families and went on to produce their own children in similar circumstances. Others managed to escape, although it proved to be impossible to generalize why. (One side-effect of this disappointing lack of hard evidence either to support or refute the transmitted deprivation hypothesis, after so much effort, was that the Social Science Research Council had 'science' removed from its title!)

Over subsequent years there was increasing criticism of the implicit 'victim blaming' ethos which lay behind the transmitted deprivation hypothesis. Researchers began to identify that individuals' behaviour is frequently conditioned by the lack of *choice* which they are able to exert over their life circumstances (Graham 1984, Blackburn 1991). At the same time research on the persistence of poverty has drawn attention to the problems of recommending healthy life styles which are beyond the material resources of many individuals and families (Burghes 1980, Lang et al 1984).

*Selective social mobility* or *selective drift* sees ill-health as the cause of poverty and deprivation. In this type of explanation the direction of causation is the reverse of that assumed in the structural and cultural explanations. Ill-health is the independent or causative variable; and poverty, unemployment and deprivation are the outcomes of ill-health (the dependent variables). In explaining the relationship between poor health and occupational class, it is argued that ill-health causes people to be downwardly socially mobile – to drift into the lower social classes. For example, if someone becomes physically or mentally ill, they might lose their job and this might result in their drifting down the social scale.

*Natural selection* is a particular variant of theories of selective social mobility. Like other selection theories it argues that ill-health causes downward mobility. In theories of natural selection the cause of the ill-health which causes downward drift is held to be genetic. The proponents of this explanation argue that people's health (physical and mental), as well as their intelligence, are the outcome of genetic factors. Differences in genetic or inherited potential determine their propensity to disease and their differing life chances.

Since the publication of the *Black Report* and *The Health Divide* the genetic base for many diseases is becoming better understood and for this reason it is important to look in some depth at these natural selection explanations which rely on differences in inherited or genetic potential. While most of the practical examples for the explanation come from developments in biochemistry and genetics, interesting theoretical perspectives may be found in the work of biosocial theorists, for example, Mascie-Taylor (1990).

It has been recognized for many years that chromosomal disorders such as trisomy 21 in Down's syndrome or genetic recessive disorders such as cystic fibrosis result from genetic factors that ultimately influence individuals' life chances and opportunities for health and, ultimately, life expectancy. Again, we would suggest that the policy implications of this explanation can be seen as 'weak' and 'strong'. The 'weak' implications can be seen in any routine screening service such as antenatal check-ups, cervical cytology, and school or occupational medical examinations. The 'strong' form lies in an as yet undeveloped potential, through genetic screening at birth, for the identification of each individual's potential life chances. In terms of health needs assessment, the possible future scenario exists where individuals' life chances such as access to education, life insurance, and various forms of employment might be determined more by their predisposition (or not) to certain diseases than by current systems of chance and opportunity. Thus the ethics of health policies which on face value appear to be benevolent carry, in theory, a potential maleficence.

Natural selection in its purest form is a bleak explanation. It leaves no place for individual or collective initiative and motivation to overcome adverse life chances. Policies directed solely at screening, counselling and medical interventions (including therapeutic abortion) leave no room for social intervention. In its most extreme form the explanation lies at the basis of eugenics theories and as such formed the sickening rationale for the National Socialists' idea of a 'master race' during the 1930s and 1940s. The potential currently exists therefore, through the development of the human genome project, for a new system of social stratification to evolve, based on individuals' genetic profiles. It seems to us that there is a strong case for arguing that the ethical implications of health needs assessment policies which enable an individual's genetic profile at birth (and therefore their life chances) to be determined, should be much more widely discussed.

### Explaining inequalities in health: discussion

It must be stressed that the above explanations (with the exception of artefact explanations) are not alternative explanations, and that the factors which give rise to ill-health frequently interact and compound one another. For example, it is known that people in poor health suffer not only from poverty and deprivation, they also tend to smoke more than those in the higher classes. The explanation for their poor health might lie not only in structural factors, but also in their health damaging behaviour. (This is not to 'blame the victims'. It is rather to point out that structural and cultural factors often combine to bring about poor health.) Similarly, it is known that poor health causes unemployment (selective drift) *and* that unemployment causes poor health (structural explanation). There is known to be a genetic component in a number of diseases, but it is also known that this cannot explain great differences in the health and social class of people with a very similar genetic endowment.

## Historical origins of contemporary inequalities in health

Finally, in attempting to understand the causes of inequalities in health it is important to be aware not only of causative factors in the recent past, but also of the historical dimension. Factors which are now known to be associated with poor health and premature death may not exert an influence until long after they have initially been experienced, as the following case study illustrates.

## CASE STUDY 2

*Inequalities in Health in Britain: Specific Explanations in Three Lancashire Towns,* Barker & Osmond (1992)

The complex relationships between the economic development of an area and its geographical features have been traced in a study of three adjacent and socially similar Lancashire towns with historic and contemporary differences in their health records. The study offers as an hypothesis the explanation that *excess* deaths from ischaemic heart disease, chronic bronchitis, stroke and bronchitis, occurring in Burnley residents at ages 55–74 years, between 1968 and 1978, can be traced back to environmental influences around the time of birth. The authors claim that their detailed historical research demonstrates that half a century before these deaths occurred, environmental influences (such as poor housing, overcrowding and less propensity to breast feed) were found in Burnley but did not predominate in neighbouring Nelson which, during 1968–78, had a mortality rate for all causes equal to the national average. In commenting on this interesting hypothesis, Klein (1991, p. 179) observes that 'it offers a warning against attempts to explain health inequalities exclusively in terms of *recent* changes in the socio-economic environment: the reasons for the inequalities may be found less in the record of the present Government than in the performance or failures of its predecessors'.

It is salutory to contemplate that the ultimate outcomes of the health promotion and prevention activities carried by a range of health care professionals, including those in the maternal, child and school health services might be found in the numbers of avoidable, premature deaths occurring half a century later. This situation clearly raises major challenges in ensuring the satisfactory audit of current community services.

## Policies to address inequalities in health

In discussing policies to deal with inequalities in health Whitehead (1995) differentiates between four layers at which influence can be exerted. Policies can be directed towards:

- strengthening individuals;
- strengthening communities;
- improving access to essential facilities and services;
- encouraging macro-economic and cultural change.

At the first level, policy responses consist of 'person-based strategies' to strengthen the individual. These include strategies such as stress management education, counselling people who have become unemployed to prevent a decline in their mental health, and smoking cessation clinics. They include also preventive and screening services. Many of the interventions which take place at this level are concerned with maternal and child health, relying on midwives, health visitors and other community nurses. Such strategies may have a direct effect on inequalities in health, for example if they decreased the prevalence of smoking in socio-economically disadvantaged groups in society, or increase the rate of uptake of immunization services among disadvantaged sections of society.

The second level is concerned with how people in disadvantaged communities can join together in ways which strengthen their resistance to health hazards. It is concerned with fostering the strengths of families, communities and voluntary associations to create healthier conditions for disadvantaged communities. At this level community development strategies have a role. An example of an intervention at this level is the traffic calming scheme introduced in Nottingham where roads which were accident 'black spots' were re-designed with 'sleeping policemen' in order to slow vehicles. Members of the community identified the need for such a scheme to reduce accident rates, and with the aid of local community workers including the police, health visitors and general practitioners, the scheme was introduced. Similar achievements by local communities have been documented in many other parts of the country (Whitehead 1995).

The third policy level described by Whitehead (1995) is about improving access to what WHO call 'the prerequisites for health' or what Doyal and Gough refer to as 'intermediate needs' (see Ch. 2). They include some of the traditional public health measures to improve access to clean water, sanitation, adequate housing, secure employment, adequate nutrition, and essential health and social care services. Although such policies benefit the health of the entire population, they benefit especially people living in the worst conditions and therefore have great potential to reduce inequalities in health. Policies at this level are often provided by different sectors so that 'intersectoral collaboration' is needed.

Finally, strategies at the fourth level include macro-economic policies such as taxation and labour market policies, the promotion of equal opportunities policies, as well as policies to control environmental pollution (Whitehead 1995).

Macro-economic policies which aim to alter the distribution of income and wealth between rich and poor are indirect rather than direct policies. They do not deal directly with inequalities in health but with the wider inequalities in society which give rise to health inequalities. There is a growing body of evidence to suggest that in Britain today, income differentials between the rich and the poor are growing. A recent Rowntree Foundation Report (Barclay 1995) confirmed that income inequality in the UK grew rapidly between 1977 and 1990, reaching a higher level in 1990 than has been recorded since 1949. The Rowntree Report concludes that between 1979 and 1992 the poorest 20–30% of the population failed to benefit from economic growth. Since poor health is closely related to poverty, such findings suggest that the inequitable distribution of income, wealth and power in society must be tackled if there is to be a reduction in inequalities in health. Wilkinson (1992, 1994) and Power (1994) argue that measures such as reducing income differentials through redistributive taxation and benefit measures, and reducing unemployment, will have an important impact on reducing inequalities in health.

## The equitable distribution of health care resources

We saw above that the *Black Report* drew attention not only to inequalities in health, as expressed in mortality and morbidity rates, but also to inequalities in access to high quality health care between different social classes. In this section we look at the question of reducing unacceptable inequalities in access to health care.

The idea of 'equal health for equal need' – that everyone with the same need for health care should have the same access to the same treatment, irrespective of their financial means or any other factor unrelated to their health need is a fundamental equity principle of the NHS (Le Grand 1987). However, developments taking place within the NHS since the publication of the *Black Report* have, in the eyes of many commentators, undermined this principle. One such development is the recently implemented NHS and Community Care Act (Department of Health 1990) which involves a transfer of responsibility for the continuing care of some elderly people by the NHS into the private sector, with some funding from the social security budget. The effect has been that some patients receive not a free service but a means tested one (Whitehead 1994). The Act is discussed in Case Study 3.

## CASE STUDY 3

The headline 'Cradle to grave NHS buried by Government' appeared in a British newspaper, *The Independent*, on Saturday, 13 August, 1994 (p. 1). This item reported draft Government guidance to health authorities, enabling them to draw up their own local definitions of who, among the elderly, is to be entitled to continuing NHS care. While welcomed by some commentators as underlining that authorities could not in future make a decision to provide *no* care, others were concerned that a major principle underlying the establishment of the NHS (namely equal entitlement to free treatment for all in need) was being eroded. Significantly for those working in the NHS, the guidance indicates that the responsibility for multi-disciplinary assessment will lie (under the terms of the NHS and Community Care Act, 1990) with Local Authorities, who may decide to purchase places in private nursing homes subject to individuals being dependent on means-tested financial support.

In its guidance, the Government is not denying that there may be a need for continuing care among the elderly, but in future neither its definition, nor the means for meeting that need, will rest solely with the NHS. This raises equity issues of particular importance to nurses for the guidelines refer specifically to medical conditions in which no further improvement can be anticipated; an area where nursing, historically, has had a major part to play. A duty of care remains, but the cost of discharging that duty must be identified and met outside the NHS either by the patient themselves or by the Social Security system. These conditions do not apply equally to other users of the NHS who may be younger, or suffering from conditions which, because of their temporary nature, can be expected to be resolved by following a reasonably clearly defined protocol for care. This suggests that the principle of equity in terms of access to free health care for everyone in need for care has been abandoned in favour of an implicit principle that only those who are likely to be cured, qualify.

The NHS and Community Care Act thus raises important questions about the lack of entitlement of old and vulnerable people to free NHS care, and questions of equity between those being treated within the NHS and those being treated in the community (Whitehead 1994). Far from promoting equity, many commentators have suggested that the Act introduces many inequities: between different client groups (those with curable conditions and those with incurable conditions), between different income groups (those who can afford to pay for continuing care and those who cannot), between those living in different localities; and, in particular, between the different generations (Challis & Henwood 1994, Judge & Mays 1994).

## Horizontal and vertical equiity

In considering ways of putting into practice the principle that access to services should be in relation to need, economists' ideas about *horizontal* and *vertical* equity are helpful. Horizontal equity expresses the idea of equal treatment for equals. Vertical equity is about unequal treatment for unequal need (Black 1994, pp. 22, 23):

> In essence, horizontal equity accords equal treatment to equals; and vertical equity give unequal, but appropriate, treatment to individuals or groups who are 'unequal' in specified respects, thereby meriting different provision.

> In the context of health care, horizontal equity could be regarded as equal access to what is available, vertical equity as the apportionment of care in relation to need.

The principles of horizontal and vertical equity are far from straightforward. Their application depends upon the way in which people are defined as 'equal' or 'unequal'. Black suggests that people are often defined as equal when, in fact, they are unequal. For example, he argues that everyone might be defined as equal in his or her entitlement to receive health education advice, and therefore the principle of horizontal equity should be applied when giving health education advice. However, Black suggests, if the circumstances of people's lives differ in such a way that one group of people is more able to act upon that advice than another, then the two groups are not in any real sense equal. Those whose circumstances make it hard for them to act upon that advice are 'unequal' and merit special attention. In this situation it is vertical equity – discrimination in favour of those less able to take advantage of services – which should be the guiding principle (Black 1994). Most economists reject Black's interpretation of vertical equity, arguing that the health service is not in the business of attempting to compensate for inequalities which arise from 'social' factors rather than strictly 'health' factors. However, many non-economists endorse Black's view, arguing that vertical equity (in the way in which Black understands it) should be an important guiding principle in the allocation of health care resources.

## CONCLUDING SUMMARY

There exist widespread inequalities in health status and in access to health care between different geographical regions, between different socio-economic classes, between different income groups, between different age groups and between those suffering different types of illness. Many inequalities in health status can only be dealt with through wide societal measures to reduce the social inequalities which give rise to health inequalities. Tackling inequalities in access to health services requires that a just or equitable means of allocating health care resources is found which does not discriminate against those unable to pay for treatment, the elderly and disabled, the poor, and other disadvantaged groups.

In this chapter we have focused on the interaction between health and inequality, and have stressed that policy must attempt to redress inequalities in health, and inequities in the distribution of health care resources. In the following chapter we look in some depth at the discipline of epidemiology, a discipline which, like sociology, emphasizes the importance of the wider social determinants of health.

# Epidemiological approaches to health needs assessment

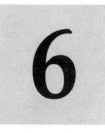

## INTRODUCTION

In Chapter 4 we examined the government's approach to health needs assessment which relies heavily on the discipline of epidemiology. In this chapter we explore in more depth epidemiological concepts and theories and their application to health needs assessment.

The chapter discusses the scope and objectives of epidemiology, and its relevance to health needs assessment. The main measuring tools employed by epidemiologists are described and the methods they rely on are discussed.

## ORIGINS AND DEFINITIONS OF EPIDEMIOLOGY

The word epidemiology is derived from the Greek. It means 'studies upon people'. Epidemiology studies *populations* rather than individuals. Epidemiology has been defined as 'the study of the distribution and determinants of health and disease frequencies in populations, for the purpose of promoting wellness and preventing disease' (McMahon & Pugh 1970, Clemen-Stone et al 1987).

Although epidemiology did not become an established discipline until the 20th century, epidemiological reasoning and methods go back to ancient times. The ancient Greek physician, Hippocrates wrote in 'On Airs, Waters and Places' that the physician should investigate matters such as the climate and geographical situation of a locality, the waters that the inhabitants use and 'the mode in which the inhabitants live, and what are their pursuits, whether they are fond of drinking and eating to excess, and given to indolence, or are fond of exercise and labour' (Hippocrates, quoted by Friedman 1985).

In more recent times epidemiology has been defined by its objective which, in the late 19th and early 20th century, was the study of epidemics of infectious diseases. This is no longer its main focus of interest. Although most epidemiological texts refer to the subject matter of epidemiology as disease, the term can be interpreted widely to include disabilities, chronic as well as acute conditions; psychiatric illnesses and events such as schizophrenia and suicide; and social problems such as drug abuse, alcoholism or child abuse (Holland & Karhausen 1978, Ryan 1983).

## Epidemiological models of disease causation

Very few diseases have only a single cause. Most of the diseases studied by epidemiologists have multiple causes. For example, tuberculosis is caused not merely by the tubercle bacillus. Although exposure to the tubercle bacillus is necessary for an individual to develop tuberculosis, it is not a suffficient cause because not everyone exposed to the tubercle bacillus gets tuberculosis. Other factors, including poverty, overcrowding, poor nutrition and alcoholism have all been identified as contributory factors which help to explain why the organism causes disease in some people but not in others (Friedman 1980). It is thus immediately apparent that effective services to deal with tuberculosis include more than narrow medical services. Measures to deal with poverty and poor housing conditions will do much to prevent this, and many other, diseases (See also final section 'Epidemiology and the health of the population').

Most of the diseases and problems in which epidemiologists are interested are the result of complex, multiple causes. One way of viewing these multiple causes is in terms of the classic triangle of *agent*, *host* and *environment*. In the case of tuberculosis the *agent* is the tubercle bacillus. When looking at the agent, factors such as the pathogenicity of the organism are important. *Host* factors are concerned with susceptibility. The extent of individual or population immunity is a factor here. Sometimes such host factors as a constitutional or hereditary pre-disposition or resistance are also important. *Environmental* factors include social conditions such as poverty, poor housing and unemployment. They also include such factors as the air quality, as well as conditions beyond human control such as the climate and the changing temperature and humidity associated with seasonal change.

Although the *agent/environment/host* triangle is usually applied to the infectious diseases with which traditionally epidemiology has been concerned, the triangle can be adapted and applied to other types of disease or problem such as cancers, accidents, or mental illness.

Another way of conceptualizing the complex train of events which leads to disease is as a *web of causation*. Heart disease, in which one set of factors leads to another, eventually resulting in a heart attack, can be viewed as the result of a web of causation. A range of factors from genetic predisposition and stress, to smoking, lack of exercise and a fatty diet, through to high blood pressure and a furring-up of the arteries, all interact and eventually result in overt disease (Friedman 1980).

Most of the physical, social and psychological problems which nurses encounter today have multiple and complex causes (Ryan 1983). For example, Finnegan & Ervin (1989) suggest that a high infant mortality rate in a particular community is related to a range of factors, including low family income, low educational level, smoking, drug use, insufficient prenatal care, teenage births, and a high rate of low-birth-weight babies. Physical illnesses such as cancer and heart disease, psychological and psychiatric disturbances, and social problems such as child abuse are all the result of the interaction of multiple factors (Ryan 1982).

# THE OBJECTIVES OF EPIDEMIOLOGICAL STUDY

## Descriptive and analytic epidemiology

A primary aim of epidemiology is accurate description. Descriptive epidemiology involves population surveys in which the amount and distribution of disease in various major subgroups of the population, or in populations of different countries, is measured and compared (Farmer & Miller 1991). A distinction can be drawn between *descriptive* and *analytic* epidemiology. Analytic epidemiology is a more focussed study of the determinants or causes of disease. The focus of analytic epidemiology is on the causes of, or reasons for, relatively high or low frequencies of disease in particular sub-groups of the population, or in different populations.

In practice the distinction between descriptive and analytic epidemiology is blurred. Large-scale descriptive studies often provide much preliminary evidence about causes, while analytic studies may fail to pinpoint causes (Friedman 1980). For example, large-scale descriptive studies of Japanese people who have migrated to the United States have found that Japanese women migrants experience a similar incidence of breast cancer to indigenous American women, and a much higher incidence than that experienced by women who remain in Japan (Friedman 1980, 1985). This is a descriptive observation but it suggests immediately that the causes of breast cancer are unlikely to be purely genetic. It suggests that there must be some environmental differences between Japan and the USA, such as perhaps dietary differences, which explain this finding. The purpose of analytic studies of breast cancer is to try to narrow down the range of possible causes.

One way to view epidemiology is as a series of steps from the description of the disease and all the factors associated with it, to hypotheses about causal agents, to the ultimate identification of the cause(s). Valanis (1986), an American Public Health Nurse, in *Epidemiology in Nursing and Health Care*, describes epidemiology in this way (Valanis 1986, p. 3):

> .... In practical terms, (epidemiology) is the study of how various states of health are distributed in the population and what environmental conditions, life styles, or other circumstances are associated with the presence or absence of disease. Epidemiologists are essentially medical detectives concerned with the who, what, where, when, and how of disease causation. By searching to find who does and who does not get sick with a particular disease and determining where the illness is and is not found, under what particular circumstances, epidemiologists narrow down the suspected causal agents. When an agent is finally identified, public health officials can take steps to prevent or control the occurrence of the disease.

## The role of epidemiology in health needs assessment

Epidemiology is central to health needs assessment. We saw in Chapter 4 that an important aim of health needs assessment is to ensure that services are reaching all those who could benefit from them. Descriptive epidemiological studies which measure the incidence and prevalence of a health problem provide information about the extent to which health problems are being missed by health care services. Such studies often highlight a large number of previously undetected problems. For example, it has been established through epidemiological study that many patients with angina never consult a doctor (Smith 1991b). Descriptive epidemiology can thus draw attention to the iceberg of problems which are not currently being dealt with by health services. In this respect epidemiology is very much concerned with the aim of promoting horizontal equity, that is, the aim of promoting equal access to what is available. It is clearly inequitable that only those whose problems are known about should have access to health-care services.

Descriptive epidemiological studies are also central to the aim of promoting vertical equity, that is, the aim of ensuring that resources are targeted on those in greater need. This is because such studies look at the distribution of disease in different sub-groups of the population. For example, a descriptive epidemiological study might compare rates of heart disease in people in different occupational classes, or in different geographical areas, or in people of different ethnic origins. Such studies are able to identify groups at particular risk so that these people can be targeted by both treatment and preventive services (Friedman 1980, Finnegan & Ervin 1989).

Information about the causes of health problems is also important for health needs assessment. An understanding of the causes of a problem provides information about whether the problem is likely to get bigger or smaller. For example, if it is known that cigarette smoking is a major cause of heart disease then information about rates of smoking can be used to predict whether the problem of heart disease is likely to get bigger or smaller. Moreover, an understanding of causes is vital to any strategy to deal with many problems. Any attempt to reduce the incidence of heart disease which does not take into account its contributory causes is likely to have only limited success. Epidemiology looks at a wide range of causal factors, from cigarette smoking to such factors as unemployment.

Epidemiology also contributes to our knowledge about the effectiveness of health care interventions. As we have seen, evaluating the effectiveness of health care is an important aspect of health needs assessment because the population's ability to benefit from health care depends on the effectiveness of that care (see Chs 2 and 4). Epidemiological methods are well suited to evaluating medical and nursing interventions, and much epidemiology is about evaluating the effectiveness of interventions designed to treat or prevent disease.

For example, epidemiological studies have been carried out to look at the effectiveness of vaccination programmes, or to assess the effectiveness of adding fluoride to water supplies (Friedman 1980).

## Measures used by epidemiologists

It is important to have some understanding of the ways in which epidemiologists measure the amount of disease or other health problems. This section looks at the main measuring tools employed by epidemiologists.

## Counts, proportions and rates

### Counts

The most simple measurement in epidemiology is a count of the number of cases of a particular condition in a given population.

### Proportions and rates

Proportions tell us more than counts because the count of cases is expressed in relation to the whole population under investigation. It is important to express counts in relation to the whole population if the count is to be meaningful and to allow for comparisons between different populations. In order to convert a count of, say, the number of university students with influenza into a proportion of the entire student population of one university it is necessary to use a *denominator*. The whole population of students at one university is the denominator. The count of students with influenza is known as the *numerator*.

The kinds of proportions used most often by epidemiologists are *rates*. Rates take the form:

$$\frac{\text{Number of students with influenza (numerator)}}{\text{Total number of students in university (denominator)}}$$

It is conventional to multiply crude rates by 100, 1000 or 10000. By multiplying the above crude rate by 100, the rate can then be stated as 'so many cases of influenza per 100 students in the university', for example 2 per 100 or 2%.

The two rates most commonly employed by epidemiologists are *prevalence rates* and *incidence rates*.

### Prevalence rates

Prevalence rates measure the number of existing cases of a disease in a defined population at one point in time or over a very short period of time such as a day. Prevalence rates can be viewed as a snapshot of an existing situation:

$$\text{Prevalence} = \frac{\text{number of } \textit{existing} \text{ cases of a disease}}{\text{total population}} \text{ at a point in time}$$

### Incidence rates

In contrast to the snapshot provided by prevalence rates, incidence rates describe the continuing occurrence of *new* cases of a disease over a defined period of time, such as a year:

$$\text{Incidence} = \frac{\text{number of } \textit{new} \text{ cases of a disease}}{\text{population at risk}} \text{ over a period of time}$$

In any kind of rate the denominator must consist of all those, and only those, who might appear in the numerator (Rose & Barker 1986). The denominator of an incidence rate is not the total population because some members of the population may not be at risk of developing the disease under investigation. Some chronic diseases last a lifetime so that those with such diseases cannot develop them again, for example, people with pre-existing diabetes. These people must be removed from the denominator.

### Period prevalence rates

The measure usually referred to as prevalence is strictly speaking *point* prevalence. There is another less common measure known as *period* prevalence. The latter measures all the disease affecting a population during a period such as a year, rather than taking a snapshot at one time. Period prevalence is made up of the prevalence at the beginning of the period (for example the start of the year 1990), plus new cases (the incidence), plus recurrences over the one year period – if one person has a recurrence of the disease under investigation then that person is counted twice.

Period prevalence rates are useful for the purposes of planning services. For example, in planning numbers of hospital beds an administrator might be interested in the one year period prevalence of cancer (Mausner & Bahn 1974).

### The relation of prevalence to incidence and duration of illness

Prevalence depends on two things: how many people have become ill in the past (i.e. the previous incidence), and the duration of their illness. If only a few people become ill each year but the disease is chronic the number will mount and the prevalence will be relatively large in relation to incidence. In the case of diseases of shorter duration, if the number of new cases (incidence) is matched by the disappearance of an equal number of existing cases (through death or recovery), then prevalence will remain at the same level. A sudden rise in the incidence of a short illness (as in epidemics of infectious diseases) is often accompanied by a rise in prevalence because the incidence of new cases outpaces the death or recovery of existing cases (Mausner & Bahn 1974, Pickin & St Leger 1994).

### Other rates: death rates and birth rates

Death rates (mortality rates) and birth rates are like incidence rates. Instead of describing the continuing occurrence of new cases of illness, mortality rates and birth rates refer to the continuing occurrence of cases of death or cases of birth respectively.

Any kind of rate can refer to a subgroup of a population. Examples are age-specific mortality rates and condition-specific mortality rates.

### Standardized mortality ratios

When comparing death rates in different populations it may be necessary to adjust the crude death rate to take into account the age and sex structure of the populations being compared. Because women have a lower mortality than men, and because mortality increases with age in both sexes, it is necessary to find a way of allowing for differences in the age and sex structures of different populations (Black 1994). One measure which allows for comparison between different populations is the standardized mortality ratio (SMR). The SMR has been defined as 'the ratio of the number of deaths actually observed in a study population to the number of deaths which would have occurred in the population if it had experienced the age-specific death rates of a standard population' (Goldacre & Vessey 1987). Thus, in essence, an SMR compares the actual death rate with the expected death rate.

Figure 6.1 illustrates the way in which Standardized Mortality Ratios have been used by Nottingham Health Authority to compare death rates between small areas within the administrative boundary of the Health Authority. A standard population would have an SMR of 100, so that an SMR above 100 indicates an excess of actual deaths over expected deaths, while an SMR below 100 indicates fewer actual deaths than would be expected.

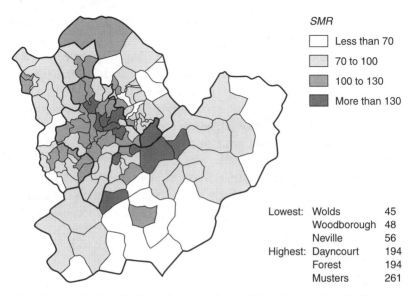

**SMR**

☐ Less than 70

▨ 70 to 100

▨ 100 to 130

▨ More than 130

| Lowest: | Wolds | 45 |
|---|---|---|
| | Woodborough | 48 |
| | Neville | 56 |
| Highest: | Dayncourt | 194 |
| | Forest | 194 |
| | Musters | 261 |

**Fig. 6.1** Nottingham Health Authority: all deaths 1984–88 (Reproduced with permission from Davies L 1990 Annual Report of the Director of Public Health 1990, Nottingham Health Authority).

## Difficulties in determining rates

The calculation of rates depends on the availability and comprehensiveness of the relevant data. Sometimes it is not possible to express a phenomenon as a rate at all. The 1992 Report on the State of the Public Health (in England) (Department of Health 1994a) reports *numbers of cases* (counts) instead of *rates* for several diseases including malaria, and HIV infection/AIDS. In the case of malaria it is difficult to determine a denominator. The denominator must consist of those, and only those, at risk of contracting malaria. The denominator for malaria cannot be the population of England since the disease is not endemic in this country, so that most people are not at risk. A valid denominator might be all those residents who have arrived in, or returned to, England from an area of the world in which malaria is endemic, but there exists no reliable record of all those persons so travelling.

In the case of AIDS and HIV infection there are difficulties in determining the numerator and the denominator. It might be thought that an appropriate denominator is the entire population of England not already suffering from AIDS – everyone is 'at risk'. However, this is not so because those people who are HIV-positive but have not yet developed AIDS are not at risk – rather they are already affected.

HIV-infected people must be excluded from the denominator and included in the numerator alongside people who have already developed AIDS. The difficulty lies in trying to identify people who are HIV-positive. There exists in England no system, such as mass screening, for identifying people with HIV infection. (We are not, of course, suggesting that mass screening should be carried out. The absence of a screening programme may impede accurate measurement, but this may be considered a small price to pay for the many advantages of not screening for HIV infection.)

Finally, it is worth noting that even a straight count of people with AIDS (or any other disease) might not be accurate because of under-reporting of the illness. Any count or a rate is only as accurate as the information on which it is based.

## Methods used by epidemiologists

### Introduction

The two broad types of epidemiology, descriptive and analytic, correspond to the different methods of study employed by epidemiologists. Of the five basic types of epidemiological methods listed below the first type (descriptive), as its name suggests, is descriptive of the general distribution of disease in a population. The remaining four methods (cross-sectional, case-control, longitudinal and experimental) are analytic. They attempt to answer specific questions or hypotheses about causes. Analytic studies often take as their starting point a descriptive finding which raises questions or suggests hypotheses that need further investigation (Friedman 1980, Ryan 1982).

The five basic epidemiological methods:

Descriptive
Case-control
Cross-sectional (prevalence)
Longitudinal
Experimental.

## Descriptive studies

Descriptive studies look at a disease or problem and relate it to a range of characteristics or variables. For example, a descriptive study might compare the incidence of a disease in men and women, in diferrent age groups, in people of differing ethnic origins, in people in different occupations, in one geographical area against another, or in one time period against another (Friedman 1985). The number of variables which can be related to the disease is infinite. As an aid to organizing the array of descriptive variables, these are conventionally classified into three types: *who* variables (who is more likely to get the disease – men or women, employed or unemployed, etc?); *place* variables (where does the disease occur most frequently?) and *time* variables (when does it occur most frequently?).

Data for descriptive studies can be obtained directly through questionnaires, interviews, home visits, or physical examinations. They can also be obtained indirectly from birth and death certificates. Routinely collected mortality and morbidity statistics are also widely used. Data can also be obtained from the census and from hospital records (Ryan 1982).

Before looking at the four remaining methods employed by epidemiologists we need to look further at the notion of causation.

## Causation and association

Descriptive epidemiology looks for associations between the disease of interest and other factors or variables. It is the strength of the statistical association between the disease and a particular variable which may give the analytic epidemiologist the first clue to a possible causal relationship. The strength of a statistical association is measured using a variety of statistical tests and the result is usually referred to in terms of its *significance*. Statistical significance is defined by the probability ($P$) that an association could be expected to occur by chance. For example, if a test shows that the association would not occur by chance more than once in a hundred times then the event is statistically significant at $P < 0.01$. If the association would not occur by chance more than 5 times out of 100 then it is statistically significant at $P < 0.05$. Strength of association is not usually accepted as significant if the association would occur by chance more than 5 times out of 100.

Vitally important though it is, statistical significance is not in itself evidence of a causal relationship. This is for several reasons. First, a statistically significant finding might be the result of chance. Statistical tests of significance tell us only that it is highly improbable that an association is a chance one, not that it is impossible. This is why a statistically significant finding in a single research study rarely suffices. Further, similar research studies might fail to find anything of statistical significance, suggesting that the results of the first study were the product of purely random fluctuations (Mausner & Bahn 1974, Friedman 1980).

Second, a statistically significant relationship between two variables might be an artefact of the research design. Bias might have crept into either the methods used to conduct the study, or the selection of the people who are being studied, so that an apparent causal relationship between two variables is in fact attributable only to artefact or bias (Mausner & Bahn 1974).

Third, an association between two variables might be entirely spurious. A rise in the birth rate in a particular village might be accompanied by the arrival of migrating storks, but this relationship is only accidental or spurious, there is little by way of a causal connection between these two events.

Fourth, an association between two variables may be indirect rather than causal. In the case of *indirect association* one variable does not cause another but rather both are related to a common, underlying or confounding variable. (Some epidemiology texts refer to indirect associations as spurious, others reserve the term spurious for associations between unconnected factors.) Much effort is expended by epidemiologists in attempting to discover whether an association between a disease and some other factor is really causal or whether the disease is due to some other confounding factor. This is because, throughout the history of epidemiology, associations which have at first appeared to be causal have later been found to be indirect, as the following example illustrates (Mausner & Bahn 1974):

In studying the statistics on deaths from cholera, William Farr, a nineteenth century Registrar General, noticed an association between cholera and altitude. Death rates from cholera were much higher in areas of low altitude where the air smelt foul, than in areas of higher altitude. Farr interpreted this as support for the then popular theory that miasma, or bad air, caused cholera. Today, we know that the areas of low altitude were also the areas where water supplies were less pure. It was the impure water, not the bad air, which led to the higher death rates from cholera. The statistical association between cholera mortality and low altitude will have looked impressive to Farr, but we now know that the two variables are only indirectly rather than causally related.

Finally, an association between two variables tells us nothing about the direction of possible causation. For example, the widely documented association between ill-health and unemployment might suggest that ill-health causes unemployment; alternatively it might suggest that unemployment causes ill-health.

It is rarely possible to prove causality through epidemiological methods, but it is possible to build up a strong case for causality. The following five criteria (Mausner & Bahn 1974, Ryan 1982) are widely used to assess the likelihood that an association between variables is causal and not spurious or indirect.

**Strength of association.** In general, the stronger the association (as measured by statistical tests of significance) the more likely that it represents a cause and effect relationship. Weak associations often turn out to be spurious or indirect.

**Consistency of association.** If an association found in one study appears in other studies with different designs and different populations, the more likely the association is to be causal (and not random or artefactual).

**Time sequence.** The characteristic or event associated with the disease must precede the disease.

**Specificity of the association.** This refers to the extent to which the occurrence of one factor or event can be used to predict the occurrence of another. The criterion is not crucial, because it is known that one factor or event can result in more than one disease and because different events or factors can result in the same disease.

**Coherence with existing information.** If a causal interpretation of an association is plausible or consistent with current knowledge, this adds support to a causal explanation. This criterion is not crucial because it depends on the state of knowledge at the time.

We can now return to the remaining four methods employed by epidemiologists.

## Cross-sectional (or prevalence) studies

Cross-sectional studies (as well as case-control studies) are an attempt to pinpoint which factors are associated with the problem under investigation. In carrying out a cross-sectional study, the study population is divided into those who have been exposed to a possible causative factor and those who have not. For example, in studying the problem of breast cancer, ths study population might be divided into those who consume a high fat diet, and those who do not; or those whose mother died of the illness, and those whose mother did not; or those whose anxious personalities are suspected of making them susceptible to cancer, and those who do not display an anxious personality. The prevalence of the disease being investigated in each of the two groups is then compared.

Prevalence studies will show whether there is an association between the suspected factor and the disease. For example, they will show whether there is an association between a high fat diet and breast cancer, or between an anxious personality and breast cancer. However, the association might not be cause-and-effect. In prevalence studies it is often difficult to determine the time sequence and thus the direction of causality. For example, if it is found that cancer sufferers exhibit more anxiety than non-sufferers, it cannot be assumed that the anxiety preceded the cancer. Cancer sufferers have good reason to feel anxious! (Friedman 1980). It may also be difficult to distinguish an indirect from a causal relationship. For example, it may be that people who consume a high fat diet also eat very little fruit and vegetables. It may be that the 'cause' is not the fat consumed but rather the absence of fruit and vegetables.

## Case–control studies

In case–control studies, individuals with the problem under investigation are matched with an equal number without the problem who are comparable in other respects such as age and sex. Data are collected from both groups about factors or attributes which are thought to be associated with the disease, such as occupation, social class, or use of alcohol or tobacco. The relative frequency of these factors in the two groups (case and control) are compared. If the cases show a higher proportion with such attributes than do the controls then there is an association between a given factor and the problem (Holland & Gilderdale 1977). The association might not be cause-and-effect. Like cross-sectional studies, case–control studies are not always able to distinguish an indirect from a causal relationship or to determine the direction of possible causality (Friedman 1980).

Case–control studies are useful not only in investigating possible causes of disease, but also in assessing the effectiveness of a health care intervention. For example, in evaluating home care nursing programmes for patients with cardiac failure, Gibson (1966) compared cardiac patients who had received nursing care in their own homes after discharge from hospital with patients who had received no home care after discharge. The relative outcomes in terms of the number of days subsequently spent in hospital were then compared, and it was shown that those who received regular home visits from nurses spent fewer days in hospital (Holland & Gilderdale 1977).

## Longitudinal studies

Longitudinal studies are prospective, unlike the three types outlined above which are retrospective. There is some confusion about the terms 'prospective' and 'retrospective'. It might be thought that cross-sectional studies such as the study of home care provided by nurses described immediately above is prospective. This study was in fact retrospective because it was undertaken after patients had received either home care or no home care. A similar study conducted prospectively would have begun before it was known which patients were to receive home care and which were not.

By studying a population over a period of time, the aim of longitudinal studies is to define the factor(s) concerned with the development of a disease or problem. It is important to undertake longitudinal studies when other types of study are unable to distinguish which of two associated factors came first.

The study undertaken by Morris et al (1994), which looked at premature death among unemployed men, is an example of this method. These investigators followed a sample of men over a period of more than 10 years. By beginning the study before any of the men in the sample had became unemployed this study was able to demonstrate not only an association between unemployment and ill health (as measured by premature death), but also the direction of causation. The research team found causality in both directions, that is, some of the unemployed men who died prematurely had lost their jobs because they were ill. However, for others, unemployment had come first and was followed by premature death. After adjustment for likely confounding variables such as social class and smoking, the findings still suggested that, for some men, unemployment was one determinant of premature death. Even in longitudinal studies, however, it can still be difficult to establish causation. The researchers could not rule out the possibility that the association they found between loss of employment and increased mortality was indirect rather than causal, i.e. that there was some other confounding factor (which would have to be closely associated with unemployment) which they had failed to identify which had given rise to the association of unemployment with premature mortality. The evidence against a causal interpretation in this study was that the increased mortality of unemployed men was from both cancer and heart disease, i.e. the effect was not specific (see above criteria for assessing causality). The researchers were at a loss to explain why mortality from cancer should be affected by loss of employment during such a short follow-up (mortality was measured on average 5.5 years after the men had become unemployed). The research team's findings were not consistent with our current knowledge about the length of time it takes to develop cancer.

## Experimental studies

Experimental studies differ from case–control studies in that they are always prospective. The exemplar of the experimental method is the controlled clinical trial. The study population is divided into two, matched groups. One group (the experimental group) receives the intervention or action or treatment under investigation, the other (the control group) does not. Experimental studies are believed to be the best test of a cause-and-effect relationship. The outcome of the intervention in the experimental group is presumed to be the effect of that intervention, provided the same outcome did not occur in the control group (Friedman 1980).

It is not always possible to carry out experimental studies, particularly in the field of nursing, for ethical reasons. For example, it would not be ethical to prescribe certain medications to an experimental group of patients solely for the purpose of establishing whether this led to their experiencing more falls than patients not taking this medication. In this instance, other methods, such as the case–control method, must be found (Ryan 1983).

Experimental studies are usually contrived in the sense that they involve some kind of manipulation on the part of the investigator. However, on rare occasions experimental conditions occur naturally: that is, two groups exist who are similar in every respect, except for their exposure to the one factor which is suspected to be a cause. The most famous example of a 'natural experiment' was that carried out in 1855 by a doctor, John Snow. Snow – and many others at the time – rejected the idea that cholera was caused by 'bad air' or miasma. Snow formulated the hypothesis that cholera was transmitted by contaminated sewerage discharged into water supplies, and this explained why some parts of London were more affected than others. It so happened that people living in the same general area of south London were served by two different water companies who drew their supplies of water from different points of the river Thames. One company's water (the company which supplied the Broad Street pump) was contaminated by sewerage from a part of London where there had recently been a cholera outbreak, the other's was not. Snow (1855, quoted in Mausner & Bahn 1974, p. 94) reported that nature had devised an

> ..... experiment... on the grandest scale (in that) no fewer than three hundred thousand people of both sexes, of every age and occupation, and of every rank and station, from gentlefolks down to the very poor, were divided into two groups without their choice, and, in most cases, without their knowledge; one group being supplied with water containing the sewerage of London, and, amongst it, whatever might have come from the cholera patients, the other group having water quite free from such impurity ..... To turn this grand experiment to account, all that was required was to learn the supply of water to each individual house where a fatal attack of cholera might occur.

Snow subsequently found an 8-fold difference in the cholera death rates for the households supplied by the two companies, giving clear evidence of an association between death from cholera and the source of water supply to the household (Mausner & Bahn 1974).

## Epidemiology and the health of the population

Throughout history, epidemiological observations have been acted upon long before there was any precise understanding of the detailed mechanisms of disease causation. John Snow's observation of a strong association between contaminated water and cholera resulted in public health measures to improve water supplies and sanitation in the absence of any knowledge at the time of the 'germ theory of disease' and the precise role of the cholera vibrio in causing cholera. Today, the precise mechanisms by which smoking gives rise to many diseases are far from fully understood, but the strong association documented in a number of epidemiological studies between smoking and premature mortality from a number of diseases has been enough to justify the policy aim of reducing smoking rates.

Epidemiological study has shown time and again that medical interventions, based on medical knowledge, have had only a limited impact on the health of the population (Friedman 1980). That medical interventions are by no means the only influence on health is illustrated by the long-term trends in mortality from many infectious diseases, such as tuberculosis or whooping cough. In the USA, Winkelstein (1972) demonstrated that mortality rates for tuberculosis had declined as a result of the amelioration of many adverse social conditions long before the introduction of effective chemotherapy (Friedman 1980). Similarly in Britain, McKeown & Lowe (1966) have shown that by the time that drug therapy and immunization for whooping cough became available, the whooping cough mortality rate had already dwindled. McKeown (1979) has convincingly shown that it has been measures such as clean water supplies and sanitation, improved nutrition (which increases resistance to disease), and improved housing conditions which have brought about the most dramatic declines in mortality (Black 1994).

Epidemiology places the role of curative medicine and nursing into perspective. It emphasizes that we cannot rely solely on effective curative interventions to improve the nation's health. The epidemiological approach underlines the fact that improvements in health are the result of interventions on a wide range of fronts, from changes in personal behaviour to changes in the physical and social environment.

In the following chapter we look at the discipline of economics in which the emphasis is on investigating the costs and benefits of alternative health care interventions.

# Economics, utilitarianism and health needs assessment

# 7

## INTRODUCTION

The discipline of health economics (which is simply the application of economic principles and methods to the subject of health) has much to contribute to health needs assessment because of its central concern with the question of how to allocate scarce resources. Any theory which appears to offer to government and purchasing authorities – such as District Health Authorities – rational solutions to the problem of an apparently limitless demand for health care in the face of finite resources has understandable appeal. The appeal of economics lies in its proposition that economic methods are the most rational and appropriate methods for determining how health care resources should be distributed. However, the economic approach is not without its critics. Some allege that economic solutions can be inequitable – they can increase rather than reduce inequalities in health. Other critics point to the way in which economic solutions can be unjust. They can result in unfair solutions to the problems of how to allocate scarce health care resources. Finally, the utilitarian ethical basis of the economic approach is rejected by many who abide by deontological ethical principles. Deontologists believe that every person's life is of equal intrinsic value, and that it is neither possible, nor ethical, to place a greater value on one person's life than another's (Seedhouse 1993). The economic notion that it may be necessary to treat one person in preference to another because this represents a more efficient use of health care resources is anathema to deontologists who believe that the health professional's 'duty of care' to each individual patient overrides any other consideration.

In Section 1 of this chapter we describe economic concepts and economic methods for weighing up the costs and benefits of health care interventions. In Section 2 we look more closely at the utilitarian ethical basis of the economic approach, and contrast it with an alternative ethical theory, deontology.

## SECTION I: APPRAISING ALTERNATIVE USES OF RESOURCES

### Introduction

Economists take as their starting point the fact that resources are scarce and hence choices must be made about their use. Economists stress that however much we expand the resources devoted to health care, for example by increasing government expenditure on the NHS, they will never be sufficient to pay for everything that could be done, and it will therefore always be necessary to choose what to leave undone. 'Every choice involves a sacrifice' said Kierkegaard (quoted by Smith 1991b). The discipline of economics is based on a recognition that if resources are finite it is not possible to do one thing without forgoing the opportunity to do something else. The lost opportunity to do something different is known in economic jargon as the *opportunity cost*. For example, the opportunity cost of devoting £1 million to neonatal intensive care is the lost opportunity to use this same sum to fund adult intensive care – or any other service.

The role of the economist is to analyse the costs and benefits of pursuing one course of action as compared to other courses of action in order to make the best use of limited resources. For economists, the 'best' use of resources is that which generates the greatest possible benefit to society as a whole at the least cost. Economists are thus concerned with *maximizing benefits (gains) from available resources* (Drummond 1978). If economists employed the language of need (which many do not – see Ch. 2) then health economics would be a question of maximizing the amount of need which can be met from available resources. Thus the criterion used by economists for deciding on the best use of resources is *efficiency*. Efficiency is about getting the most out of available resources. It is about 'value for money'.

Economists do not regard themselves as qualified to make decisions about what ought to be the ultimate goals of health care. These are not economic decisions. For example, economists cannot decide whether it is more important to improve the quality of life of children with disabling but non life-threatening diseases, or whether it is more important to reduce mortality among elderly people. Such decisions invariably involve ethical and political considerations. Economists claim to work within society's 'preferences'. Once societal decisions have been arrived at about what are the desired outcomes of health care, then economists see their role as trying to find the best way of achieving them, by comparing the costs and benefits of pursuing these outcomes through different health care interventions. Of course matters are not this simple. 'Society' never does arrive at a consensus about its preferences – about what goals or outcomes are desirable and should be pursued. This is always a political matter of competing views, and economists are not above the fray of competing values and viewpoints in society. However, health economists do not lay down the law about what specific goals should be pursued. The ultimate political and ethical questions of which kinds of outcomes are the most valued and should be pursued, economists claim to leave to others.

## Economic evaluation

Economists employ three main techniques to compare the costs and benefits of health care interventions: cost–benefit analysis, cost-effectiveness analysis and cost–utility analysis (see Drummond et al 1994).

### Cost–benefit analysis

Cost–benefit analysis is a technique which makes it possible to compare the costs of a health care intervention with its benefits by expressing both costs and benefits in monetary terms. An example of a cost–benefit study is Helliwell and Drummond's (1988) study of the costs and benefits of preventing influenza among elderly people in Ontario, Canada. In this study, the costs to the Ministry of Health in Ontario of running its immunization programme were determined by adding together the costs of producing, distributing and administering the vaccine, as well as the costs of treating side-effects. Costs amounted to $1 337 700, or $7.54 per immunization. The benefits which were considered were the avoidance of hospitalization, and the physician and prescription costs averted by preventing influenza in the elderly. Benefits were valued at $2 021 267 – or $11.40 per immunization. The net benefit of the immunization programme was thus $683 567 ($2 021 267 minus $1 337 700).

In cost–benefit analysis, the expression of all cost and benefits in monetary terms does necessarily mean that only financial costs and benefits are considered. In the above example, only direct financial costs and benefits were considered. However, in many cost–benefit studies, non-monetary costs and benefits are also taken into consideration and translated into financial terms. For example, it would be possible to carry out a study of the costs and benefits of preventing influenza in elderly people which included what economists term 'intangible' costs and benefits. Intangible costs would be the loss of health status suffered by those elderly people in whom the vaccine had produced side-effects. The intangible benefits of the immunization programme would be that it had averted pain, suffering and possibly death in elderly people. Where cost–benefit studies take into consideration such 'intangibles' a monetary value must be placed upon them.

Although cost–benefit analysis is the oldest and most influential form of economic appraisal its application to the field of health care is problematic because it is so difficult, and many believe inappropriate, to place a monetary value on all the costs and benefits of health care. It is acknowledged by many economists that the process of placing a monetary value on all of the costs and benefits of health care is complex, arbitrary, and ultimately unsatisfactory. One solution to this problem is to stick measuring those costs and benefits which are most easily translated into monetary terms – as did Helliwell and Drummond in their study of immunization against influenza. Yet this is to ignore the most important benefits of health-care interventions, namely their *health* benefits. It is because of this difficulty of attaching monetary values to health benefits that cost–benefit analysis has been abandoned by many health economists in favour of cost–utility analysis, where benefits are not expressed in monetary terms (see below).

Despite its shortcomings, even those who are most critical of cost–benefit analysis acknowledge its merits in encouraging systematic thought about all the possible costs and benefits of an intervention. In other words, the thinking behind the process of cost–benefit analysis is acknowledged to be useful, if not the actual process of placing a monetary value on all costs and benefits (see Holland 1983).

The strength of cost–benefit studies is that they enable comparisons to be made between very different types of health-care intervention. Money is the common yardstick which enables very different interventions to be compared. For example, by relying on cost–benefit studies it is possible to compare the net benefits of an influenza immunization programme with the net benefits of a programme of providing, for example, cataract operations. (This is also possible using cost–utility analysis.) By contrast cost-effectiveness analysis (discussed below) is limited to looking only at interventions with the same objectives.

### Cost-effectiveness analysis

Cost-effectiveness analysis, like cost–benefit analysis, involves comparing the costs of interventions with their benefits. In cost-effectiveness studies, as in cost–benefit studies, costs are expressed in financial terms. Benefits, on the other hand, are expressed in terms of health outcomes such as 'life-years saved' rather than in monetary terms. The aim of cost-effectiveness analysis is to determine how to achieve a single, given objective, such as saving life, at minimum cost. Thus unlike cost–benefit analysis, cost-effectiveness analysis does not involve looking at a wide range of possible outcomes or benefits. Cost effectiveness studies look only at a single, pre-determined, outcome as a measure of benefit. An example of a cost-effectiveness study is the study by Klarman et al (1968) which compared the costs and benefits of two interventions for patients with end-stage renal failure – transplantation and dialysis. These authors concluded that transplantation was the cheaper way of achieving the objective of prolonging life (Maynard 1993).

The main limitation of cost-effectiveness analysis is the fact that it looks only at a single outcome, since this restricts the comparability of interventions to those with similar objectives. Studies of cost-effectiveness do not enable comparisons and choices to be made between, for example, an influenza immunization programme and cataract surgery because in the former the measure of effectiveness which is likely to be chosen is 'life-years saved', whereas in the latter the most appropriate effectiveness measure is the 'quality of remaining life'. Similarly cost-effectiveness analysis does not enable comparisons to be made between curative cancer care and palliative cancer care because again the effectiveness measure for the two is different.

## Cost–utility analysis: QALYs

Cost–utility analysis, like both cost–benefit analysis and cost-effectiveness analysis, is an attempt to compare the costs of interventions with their benefits. In cost–utility analysis costs are measured in financial terms and benefits are measured and compared in terms of health (rather than in monetary terms). However, instead of the one-dimensional measure of outcome used in cost-effectiveness analysis, cost–utility analysis employs a two-dimensional measure of outcome which combines aspects of both quality and quantity of life. Cost–utility analysis assesses interventions in terms of their ability both to increase the length of life and enhance the quality of life. These two dimensions are combined in a single measure of outcome, the Quality Adjusted Life Year (QALY). Thus, in cost–utility analysis, a given health care intervention is assessed by comparing the cost of the intervention with its benefits in terms of QALYs. An example of a cost–utility study is a Williams' (1985a) study which looked at the costs and benefits of coronary by-pass surgery.

QALYs were devised by economists because it was recognized that much medical and nursing care is given for conditions which are not immediately life-threatening, and that therefore for some conditions, 'cure' is neither a realistic nor an appropriate objective. Economists recognized the need for an outcome measure which combined information on the quality as well as the quantity of life. Cost–utility analysis came into being as a solution to the problem of cost-effectiveness analysis that it uses only a one-dimensional measure of outcome (often 'life-years saved'), and thus cannot be used to compare interventions with differing objectives; and also as a solution to the problem of cost–benefit analysis that health benefits must be translated into monetary terms.

Those who advocate cost–utility analysis and the use of QALYs accept that they are not without problems. However, they believe that QALYs represent the best solution we have, to date, to the problem of how to compare different health states and to decide on priorities. Thus, Walker (1992), quoted by Black (1994, p: 28), believes that:

> QALYs may not be the universal calculus of health care, and using them will not result in the depoliticisation of setting priorities for health care.
> However, they represent, I believe, an important stage both of our thinking about health status, and of a common language for expressing health states.

QALYs are discussed further in Section 2.

In Chapter 8 we illustrate what is involved in thinking systematically about costs and benefits in relation to one particular type health care intervention, screening. Below we compare economic approaches to evaluation with other approaches.

## Economic evaluation and other types of evaluation

Economic techniques of evaluation (namely, cost–benefit analysis, cost-effectiveness analysis, and cost–utility analysis) consider the value both of the inputs used, that is, the resources consumed, and the outputs or outcomes produced by the interventions being evaluated. This is not true of all evaluative frameworks. Below we consider two other types of evaluation, input monitoring; and medical, epidemiological and nursing evaluation.

### Input monitoring: quantitative and qualitative

A great deal of evaluation in the health service monitors only inputs without regard to the outputs or outcomes that they produce. For example, comparisons are made of hospital costs per inpatient week, or of the costs of the services provided (Drummond 1978). Many Health Service Indicators (performance indicators) compare only inputs. Clearly it is an important shortcoming of such procedures that they are unable to relate the information gathered on the resources consumed to any results or benefits produced. This shortcoming is widely recognized. Much health service evaluation of the type undertaken by District Health Authorities relies on input monitoring for pragmatic reasons, in the absence of data which would enable inputs to be related to outcomes (see Chapters 4, 9 and 10).

As well as quantitative input monitoring, other types of more qualitative input monitoring are also much in evidence, for example, medical or nursing audit, or peer review. Such monitoring of the quality of inputs can be an indirect way of monitoring outcomes. However, economists believe that the difficulty with such approaches is the untested belief that 'good' inputs or processes result in 'good' outcomes. Without taking outcomes into consideration, the belief that 'good' inputs equals 'good' outputs cannot be put to the test (Drummond 1978).

Economists tend to view it as a failure of qualitative monitoring that inputs and processes are not related to outcomes. However, health care professionals, and particularly nurses, argue that for some interventions the outcome or output is unimportant. There are aspects of benefit which relate to the *process* of delivering health care that are independent of its outcome (Downie & Elstein 1988, Drummond 1993). For example, in providing nursing care to terminally ill patients what is all-important is the way in which care is delivered – the *process* of caring. To judge whether the process of terminal care has been successful in terms of an outcome measure such as whether the patient dies a bit sooner or a bit later is not an appropriate way of evaluating the benefits of terminal nursing care.

### Medical, epidemiological and nursing evaluation

Economic evaluation depends to some extent on other types of evaluation. Much economic evaluation requires an estimation of the medical or nursing effectiveness of health care interventions. For example, Klarman's study of the cost-effectiveness of transplantation versus dialysis for renal failure was dependent on medical knowledge about the effectiveness of these two interventions. Klarman et al needed to know how successful these two interventions were in achieving the objective of prolonging life before they could assess their cost-effectiveness. However, medical and epidemiological evaluation of the effectiveness of interventions suffers the converse problem to input monitoring. It considers only the effectiveness of interventions or treatments (outcomes) but not the value of the resources that these consume (inputs). For economists, an estimation of medical or nursing effectiveness is always necessary in deciding on the best use of resources, but this is sometimes insufficient. Where medical or nursing effectiveness studies alone might suffice for economists is where they identify ineffective treatments. This is because ineffective treatments are not cost-effective either. They consume scarce resources yet produce few benefits to society, and are therefore inefficient. However a major problem arises when, given limited resources, it is necessary to choose between alternative treatments all of which have been shown to be effective in varying degrees. If *effectiveness* is the only criterion used, then the most effective treatment is the treatment of choice from the range of alternatives. However, if *cost-effectiveness* is the criterion, then the relative costs of alternative treatments must be taken into account. It may be that when cost-effectiveness is the criterion, this will result in the selection of a less effective but also less costly treatment.

It is not the case that economists believe that cheapness is more important than effectiveness. The economists' approach is based on the fact of scarcity, the fact that all uses of resources carry opportunity costs. Economists argue that given limited resources, the extra resources consumed by the more costly (and more effective) treatment could be put to other beneficial uses.

## Efficiency versus equity

We have seen above that for economists, the best use of resources is that which maximizes benefits to *society as a whole*. However, it is sometimes the case that maximizing health benefits to society as a whole may greatly increase costs to some sections of society. For example, in comparing institutional care and 'community care' it might be found that it is community care which maximizes benefits in relation to costs, to society as a whole. However, community care policies undoubtedly increase the costs born by one section of society – informal carers. Costs to carers of 'community care' policies include first, the direct costs of providing materially for the person they are caring for; second, the intangible, emotional costs of caring; and third, indirect costs which include the time spent in caring, and perhaps also the financial costs incurred by having to give up paid employment to undertake the job of caring. For society as a whole community care might represent a more efficient use of resource, but for informal carers, costs are greatly increased in relation to benefits. Thus community care policies might be more efficient but they are not equitable. Costs are not distributed equitably between different groups in society.

Similarly, although a given health care intervention might maximize benefits to society as a whole, in so doing it might increase differences in the amount of benefit received by different groups in society – it might widen inequalities in health. For example, increased rates of uptake for screening for cervical cancer might reduce mortality from the disease in society as a whole, but since uptake rates are far lower in social classes IV and V than in higher social classes, increased rates of uptake in society as a whole may increase differences in the amount of benefit experienced by those belonging to different social classes (Reading et al 1994, see also Ch. 8).

Although economic analysis can highlight the different groups in society who bear costs and receive benefits it cannot resolve questions about the most fair distribution of costs and benefits. It cannot deal with questions of equity. For this reason, many health economists acknowledge that the economic criterion of efficiency is an inadequate basis on which to decide how best to distribute health care resources. For some economists the 'best' use of resources must be one which not only promotes efficiency but is also equitable (Williams 1993b). The notions of 'horizontal' and 'vertical' equity, which were discussed in Chapter 5, were developed by economists who recognized the limitations of relying only on the criterion of efficiency to decide how best to distribute health care resources. Equity is discussed further in Section 2.

## Summary

The economic approach can be summarized as follows (see Drummond 1978, p. 80):

1. Economists consider that the criterion of economic efficiency, which implies the use of available resources so as to generate the largest possible benefit to society as a whole at the least cost, is essential in considering the best use of resources.

2. Some economists acknowledge that equity, which implies the use of available resource to arrive at a distribution of costs and benefits which is fair or just is also important in considering the best use of resources.

3. Economists argue that economic evaluation provides a better framework for choice between alternative health care interventions than evaluation techniques which consider only inputs (input monitoring) or outcomes (medical, epidemiological and nursing evaluation).

4. Economic evaluation relies on an assessment of the effectiveness of interventions, and therefore economic evaluation depends on medical, epidemiological and nursing evaluation.

## SECTION 2: THE ETHICAL BASIS OF ECONOMIC EVALUATION

In this section we look at the ethical basis of the economic approach, and examine the implications of alternative ethical theories for allocating scarce resources.

### Utilitarianism

The economic approach is often described as utilitarian. Utilitarianism is an ethical theory which holds that ethical decisions and behaviour are based on an assessment of the likely outcomes or consequences of actions (utilitarianism is a form of 'consequentialism'. The difference between the two need not concern us.) Thus for utilitarians, to behave ethically is to strive to produce 'good' outcomes or consequences. 'Good' can, of course, be defined in different ways. In health care a 'good' outcome might be one that decreases mortality or adds to the quality of life, rather than one which promotes 'happiness' or 'pleasure'. For utilitarians it is those decisions and actions which produce the 'greatest good for the greatest number', or the 'greatest balance of good over bad', which are the most moral or ethical. Thus utilitarianism is about weighing up the consequences of different courses of action, about assessing the benefits and disadvantages of pursuing different course of action (Seedhouse 1993).

The utilitarian basis of economic evaluation will be immediately apparent. The central plank of economics is the weighing up of the costs and benefits of alternative courses of action with the aim of making choices which maximize the benefits to society. The most efficient use of scarce resources is thus, for economists, also an ethical use of resources. Economists do not deny the utilitarian basis of their approach. On the contrary, they stress the virtue of their way of proceeding (Mooney 1992, p. 19): 'It is the task of economists to "spread a little happiness" or, more accurately, to spread as much happiness as resources will permit – a laudable goal indeed'.

## The limitations of utilitarianism

The main advantage of utilitarianism is that it allows careful and rational consideration of the consequences (outcomes) of alternative courses of action. However, one major problem with all forms of utilitarianism is that 'good' is not distributed evenly or fairly. As we saw in Section 1 of this chapter it may well be that in the population as a whole, a utilitarian policy would create a greater balance of 'good' over 'bad'. However, for some groups or individual people, more 'bad' than 'good' might be created. In other words, some people may have to suffer for the benefit of the rest of the population. Seedhouse (1993) illustrates this using the following stark quotation from Raphael (Raphael 1981):

> '. . . let us imagine that the happiness of the whole human race were to be immeasurably increased – poverty eliminated . . . . disease conquered . . .

but the condition is that one man . . . is to be kept involuntarily in a state of continuous and agonising torture. According to the utilitarian criterion, which measures the rightness of an act by its results, it would seem that the argument is justified . . . . the net balance of the utilitarian moral scale would have to point in the direction of maximum happiness and away from the eternal agony of the single suffering man. But most people who consider the proposed bargain feel that there is something terribly wrong with it.'

Of course, no economist would urge that an individual be kept in 'eternal agony' for the net benefit of the rest of society. Economists would accept that any costs must be ethically acceptable to society as a whole. Keeping an individual in a state of agony is an ethically unacceptable cost. The above example illustrates that there are questions aside from utilitarian calculations of net benefits over costs which must be taken into consideration in deciding on the best use of resources. Questions concerning which kinds of costs are ethically acceptable, and which are not, cannot be ignored.

## QALYs

QALYs, which focus on the outcomes or consequences of health care interventions, are said to exemplify utilitarian principles. In this section we explore QALYs in greater depth.

### What is a QALY?

We saw in Section 1 that a QALY is an outcome measure, it is a measure of the benefit of a health care intervention. Alan Williams, one of the architects of QALYs, describes them as follows (Williams 1985b):

The essence of a QALY is that it takes a year of healthy life expectancy to be worth 1, but regards a year of unhealthy life expectancy as worth less than 1. Its precise value is lower the worse the quality of life of the unhealthy person (which is what the 'quality adjusted' bit is all about).

QALYs are thus calculated by estimating the increase in survival which a particular intervention brings about, and then modifying this to take account of any reduction in quality of life which might remain after the intervention (Black 1994). For example, if an intervention is expected to increase life expectancy by 5 years, and it is anticipated that these 5 years will be fully healthy, then this intervention generates 5 QALYs. However, if these 5 years are expected to be only 80% fully healthy, then this intervention generates $5 \times 0.8 = 4$ QALYs.

An important assumption underlying QALYs is that an extra year of healthy life is equally valuable to everybody. 'A QALY is a QALY is a QALY', no matter who is the beneficiary (Williams & Kind 1992). QALYs do not take into account whether beneficiaries are elderly or young, or whether they belong to social class I or V. QALYs are not interested in the characteristics of the individuals or groups receiving treatment, only in the outcomes of that treatment for people-in-general. It is for this reason that some economists claim that QALYs are egalitarian and represent an equitable solution to the problem of allocating scarce resources. This is discussed further below.

### What is a QALY league table?

Williams goes on to describe the thinking behind the construction of QALY league tables (Williams 1985b):

> The general idea is that a beneficial health care activity is one that generates a positive amount of QALYs, and that an efficient health care activity is one where the cost per QALY is as low as it can be. A high priority health care activity is one where the cost-per-QALY is low, and a low priority activity is one where the cost-per-QALY is high.

Interventions can thus be ranked in order of priority. Table 7.1, which uses 1983/4 prices, ranks a series of interventions in order of their cost per QALY. The table shows that, for example, it costs £700 to provide someone requiring a pacemaker with an additional year of healthy life, whereas it costs £5000 to provide someone requiring a heart transplant with an additional year of healthy life.

### How is the 'quality of life' defined and measured in a QALY?

The measurement of the 'quality of life' invariably involves value-

**Table 7.1** A QALY league table

| Intervention | Cost per QALY gained (£) |
| --- | --- |
| GP advice to stop smoking | 170 |
| Pacemaker implantation for heart block | 700 |
| Hip replacement | 750 |
| GP control of total serum cholesterol | 1 700 |
| Kidney transplantation (cadaver) | 3 000 |
| Breast cancer screening | 3 500 |
| Heart transplantation | 5 000 |
| Hospital haemodialysis | 14 000 |

Reproduced with permission from Mooney (1992, p. 45).

judgements about what is a good quality of life and what is not. Economists claim that they do not themselves make judgements about these matters but rather their role is to reflect societal preferences and value-judgements. This is what the term 'utility' is about (see Section 1, 'cost–utility analysis'). The term 'utility' refers to the value or worth of a specific health state. If individuals or society express a preference for a particular health state, if they believe a particular health state is desirable, then this is its utility.

One of the first attempts to define and measure the 'quality of life' was made by Rosser (Rosser & Watts 1972, Rosser & Kind 1978, Kind, Rosser & Williams 1982). Rosser asked 70 people – consisting of doctors, nurses, patients and healthy volunteers – to assess various health states. In Table 7.2 we reproduce Rosser's findings. Rosser's 'quality of life' index was based on the assumption that there are two components of 'quality of life': freedom from pain or distress, and freedom from 'disability'. Respondents were asked to assign 'utility values' to various health states which combined a degree of disability with a degree of pain and distress (from no pain or distress to severe pain or distress). The scores in Table 7.2 combine the valuations of all 70 respondents. A score of less than 0 is equal to 'worse than being dead'.

Other indices of 'quality of life' have since been developed, for example the 'Index of Health-related Quality of Life' (IHQL) which distinguishes between physical and emotional distress (Rosser et al 1992).

Below we discuss criticisms which have been levelled against QALYs and QALY league tables.

## Criticisms of QALYs and QALY league tables

### Quantity versus quality

We have seen that QALYs combine in a single measure aspects of both quantity and quality of life. However, some critics argue that it is not possible to compare quality with quantity because the two are conceptually different things. No-one disputes that it is a different concept to measure the duration of life than it is to measure the quality of life. What is at issue is whether it is possible to make trade-offs between the two. For example, not everyone would agree that 4 years in perfect health is the exact equivalent of 5 years of '20% less than perfect health', yet both yield a score of 4 QALYs. Some people might prefer to live longer, even if their 'quality of life' is less than perfect.

**Table 7.2** Rosser's disability/distress matrix[a]

| Disability rating | Distress rating | | | |
|---|---|---|---|---|
| | **None** | **Mild** | **Moderate** | **Severe** |
| I No disability | 1.000 | 0.995 | 0.990 | 0.967 |
| II Slight social disability | 0.990 | 0.986 | 0.937 | 0.932 |
| III Severe social disability or slight impairment of performance at work, or both, able to do all housework except heavy tasks | 0.980 | 0.972 | 0.956 | 0.912 |
| IV Choice of work or performance at work severely limited, housewives and old people able to do only light housework but able to go out shopping | 0.964 | 0.956 | 0.942 | 0.870 |
| V Unable to undertake any paid employment, unable to continue any education, old people confined to home except for escorted outings and short walks and unable to shop, housewives able to perform only a few simple tasks | 0.946 | 0.935 | 0.900 | 0.700 |
| VI Confined to a chair or wheelchair or able to move only with support | 0.875 | 0.845 | 0.680 | 0.000 |
| VII Confined to bed | 0.677 | 0.564 | 0.000 | -1.486 |
| VIII Unconscious | -1.028 | * | * | * |

[a]Source: Kind et al (1982).
1 = Healthy.
0 = Dead.
* = Inapplicable
Reproduced with permission from Hopkins A (ed) 1992 Measures of the Quality of Life. Royal College of Physicians, London

Thus, some critics believe that we should stick to measuring the duration of life because it is ethically unjustified to suggest that quantity can be traded off against quality.

## Prolonging healthy life versus a dignified death

QALYs embody the idea that we should not attempt to prolong unhealthy life, but many health care professionals point out that prolonging healthy life is not the only, nor even the most important, benefit of health care. Providing high-quality terminal care, where there is little prospect either of increasing the duration of life, or altering the patient's health status, is a very important health benefit which QALYs cannot take into account (Black 1994). Many health care professionals thus challenge the way in which QALYs give a low priority to interventions which do not attempt to prolong healthy life. This is discussed further below.

### QALY league tables and equity

It is recognized that there are dangers of relying solely on QALY league tables to determine priorities. Taken to their logical conclusion they suggest that some groups in society whose treatment has a high cost per QALY must be denied treatment. In Oregon, USA, league tables were drawn up with the ultimate intention of choosing a cut-off point below which treatments with a very high cost per QALY would not be funded (see Kirk 1993). The Oregon experience suggests that reliance on QALY league tables can lead to ethically unacceptable solutions. The selection of a cut-off point is always arbitrary to an extent. It is unacceptable to offer treatment to those who could benefit from treatments immediately above the cut-off point but not to those who need treatments which lie below the cut-off point.

An important criticism of QALYs and league tables is that they rely only on the criterion of efficiency, not on that of equity or distributive justice. As we discussed in Section 1, the criterion of equity means that a fair means should be found of distributing the benefits of health care. QALY league tables are not about the fair or equitable distribution of benefits. They can help to tell us what is the relative cost of different types of interventions and thus provide some guidance to the most efficient use of resources, but they do not tell us what is the most just or equitable distribution. For example, QALYs cannot tell us whether it is better to offer one person 10 more years of healthy life, or 10 people one more year of healthy life.

QALYs have also been said to discriminate against certain client groups, in particular the elderly, for whom there is, by definition, only very little scope for prolonging life. All treatments which are offered mainly to elderly people are likely to register a lower QALY score than treatments which are offered mainly to younger people. QALYs have also been said to discriminate in favour of those in the higher social classes. This is because some types of health care intervention, for example surgical interventions, are performed far more on people in higher social classes than those in lower social classes. For example, coronary by-pass surgery tends to be performed largely on the more affluent, in contrast to surgery for hernias which are more prevalent in manual workers. Since it is known that a population drawn from social class I is likely to respond better to many interventions (and thus register a higher QALY score) than a population drawn from the lower social classes, this could increase the QALY rating of by-pass surgery in comparison to hernia operations (Black 1994). It is precisely because QALYs fail to take account of who is the beneficiary of health care, it is because they fail to take into account the different characteristics of different sections of society, that they are inequitable. The assumption that 'a QALY is a QALY is a QALY' does not in reality mean that QALYs are a fair and equitable solution to the problem of how to distribute health care resources.

Arguably it is possible to weight QALYs in favour of the elderly and the more deprived sections of society who lose out by an unweighted measure. Alternatively, it is often suggested that QALYs should be weighted in favour of the young. Weighting, economists believe, might make QALYs more acceptable to some people as an instrument for deciding on the equitable allocation of resources (Williams & Kind 1992). However, there are some critics who believe that QALYs, however refined, could never be used as a basis for resource allocation. Such critics, as we shall see below, believe that QALYs can never adequately represent the value of life.

### The quality of life versus the value of life

Those who question whether QALYs could ever form the basis for decisions about resource allocation tend to be those who abide by deontological ethical principles. Deontologists question the ethical assumptions underpinning the very idea of measuring the quality of life. Life has a value, deontologists maintain, which has nothing to do with whether a person's functional ability is impaired, or the severity of their pain and distress. Deontologists argue that the intrinsic value of life can never be encapsulated in something called a 'quality of life' index. Deontologists thus question whether we can really say that the value of the life of someone suffering from the pain and disability of arthritis, or enduring the mental suffering and anguish of schizophrenia, is less than that of other people. Deontologists would question too whether the value of the life of, say, someone like Stephen Hawkings, the theoretical physicist, can really be judged against such indicators as 'confined to a wheelchair'. Above all, deontologists ask: who is one person to judge the value of another's life? Deontologists do not believe that economists, or health care professionals, or lay people are in any position to judge the value of another person's life. Thus, for deontologists, it is not a question of devising better indicators of the quality of life, or weighting QALYs to make them more equitable. Deontologists reject altogether the ethical basis of QALYs – the notion that an unhealthy life is of less value than a healthy life. Of course, they agree that we should do everything we can to treat treatable conditions and to relieve suffering. However, deontologists, in contrast to utilitarians, assert that life has an intrinsic value and that all people are fundamentally equal, irrespective of their state of health. 'Equal respect for every life' is the deontologists' abiding principle. This is the principle embodied in the Hippocratic oath which states that a physician's duty of care to his patient overrides any other consideration. It is a principle which is of course particularly significant for nurses who are frequently in the position of providing care for the old and sick for whom all else has failed. For nurses, the duty to provide care to each and every patient, young or old, suffering from a curable or an incurable condition, overrides any utilitarian consideration of costs per QALY.

## The allocation of scarce resources: deontology versus utilitarianism

QALYs are about rationing. They are one solution to the problem of how to decide between competing demands on scarce resources. They are a solution which is unacceptable to deontologists but they too must grapple with the question of how to ration resources.

Some deontologists assert that the only fair way to ration is to do so on a random basis. Instead of relying on value-judgements about who should receive resources at the expense of others (playing God) rationing should be conducted on the basis of chance. Hence, decisions about who to treat should be made on the basis of factors such as mere order of presentation for treatment, as for example is often the case with waiting lists (Paton 1992). Alternatively, Harris has advocated rationing by lottery (Harris 1985). For example, if there are ten critically ill patients, all of whose lives could be saved, and only one hospital intensive care bed, then lots should be drawn to decide who receives treatment (Seedhouse 1993).

Apart from its sheer impracticality, there are other objections to the 'lottery solution'. Although it is an equitable solution, it may not always be just. To appreciate why this should be so, a very brief consideration of the notion of 'justice' is in order. Seedhouse distinguishes two notions of justice: the first is contained in the expression 'to each according to what he needs'; the second in the expression 'to each according to what he deserves'. Seedhouse argues that the former is a basic principle in health care work, whereas the latter, which expresses the idea that only those who deserve to be treated through their efforts should receive treatment, is highly contentious as a basis for making decisions about health care (Seedhouse 1993). However, some might argue that the principle of 'just desert' cannot be dismissed lightly. To return to the lottery, it could be objected that if a smoker, who knew the risks of smoking, and whose illness was caused in large measure by smoking, drew the longest straw and was thus chosen above all the others to be saved, this was unjust. The smoker did not *deserve* to be given priority even though his *need* (health problem) was as great as that of the others in the lottery. There are other grounds too, aside from its injustice, for rejecting the lottery solution. Doctors and economists might argue that smokers should have lower priority for treatment for such conditions as heart disease or lung cancer, not because they are undeserving, but because treatment for these conditions is not as effective or cost-effective in smokers as in non-smokers. There are thus good grounds for questioning the deontologist's assertion that since the value of the life of a smoker is equal to the value of life of the non-smoker, they should have an equal chance of treatment.

There are other, grave objections to the idea that everyone should have an equal chance of treatment. Seedhouse (1993) describes the scenario of a doctor having to explain to a mother that her young child has been sacrificed as the result of a lottery to save an old man with only months left to live. In this instance the utilitarian's willingness to judge a young life to be more worth saving than an old life seems the less morally reprehensible approach. To refuse to discriminate between people on the grounds of age – or anything else – and thus to leave the choice of life or death to chance seems in this instance to be an inadequate way of translating into practice the principle of 'equal respect for every life'.

Finally, some economists have suggested that leaving to chance the question of who is to receive treatment may in reality turn out to favour the better-off and more vocal sections of society. Those who 'shout loudest' may be treated more preferentially than those less able to articulate their needs. Economists argue that QALYs, which rely on impartial criteria, are a preferable means of choosing who is to receive treatment than relying on the personal and subjective judgements of health care professionals, who may simply respond to the needs of those best able to articulate their demands.

To conclude, there is no solution to resource decisions in health care. Neither utilitarian nor deontological solutions seem wholly acceptable. Deontologists believe it is unethical or immoral for one person to make judgements about the value of another person's life. Economists by contrast stress that it is inevitable, given scarcity, that resources devoted to one person will deprive another who might have benefitted more from them.

## CONCLUSION

At the heart of the tensions so frequently experienced between health care practitioners and economists lies the difference between their respective objectives and guiding ethical principles. Health care practitioners are steeped in the individual ethics of duty towards each patient in their care. They stress the importance of the *process* of caring, and believe that everyone has a right to some level of care, even if that care does not increase longevity or decrease disability. By contrast economists' utilitarian approach leads them to focus only on the consequences or *outcomes* of care. They focus only on the objective of prolonging healthy life.

A further tension surrounds the goal of promoting equity. Many health care professionals believe that deprived people should be afforded better access to health care in proportion to their greater need. Economists by contrast argue that if equity is the main objective rather than efficiency, this will mean that the overall health of the population will be worse than it need have been – people-in-general will die sooner and suffer more ill-health than they need have done (Williams & Kind 1992).

Despite their differences, health care practitioners have much to learn from economists and economists from health care practitioners. Economists have taught health care practitioners that if they decide to use up scarce health care resources on one group of patients these resources are not available to other patients. Economists have taught health care practitioners that they must choose between meeting different health needs, and prioritize in the face of scarce resources. The need to weigh up costs and benefits in a rational and systematic way, and the need to set priorities, are as relevant to the day-to-day work of nurses and other health care practitioners as they are to governments or District Health Authorities.

Economists too can learn from health care practitioners. Health care practitioners have taught economists that efficiency cannot be the only criterion in deciding on the best use of resources if this discriminates against the more deprived sections of society. Health care practitioners too have stressed the importance of finding a just means of distributing health care resources. Health care professionals, unlike economists, are often in the position of justifying to patients what might appear in patients' eyes to be an unjust policy. Finally, health care practitioners have brought home to economists that health care professionals have a 'duty of care' to each and every patient which cannot be simply abandoned in favour of a policy of caring only for those patients who have the potential for a longer, healthier life.

# Screening: health needs assessment and the evaluation of services

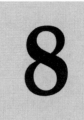

8

## ■ CONTENTS

## INTRODUCTION

In this chapter we concentrate on screening as a special example of the way in which it is possible to evaluate health care interventions. It will be clear from preceding chapters that evaluation of services is central to health needs assessment. This is because the 'ability to benefit' from health care services depends on the effectiveness of such services. We saw in Chapter 4 that evaluation studies of many health services are lacking. However, in the area of screening some evaluation has taken place, and attempts have been made to draw up criteria against which to evaluate services. This chapter discusses these criteria, and highlights a range of issues – practical, economic and ethical – which must be taken into account in evaluating screening services. Many of the issues highlighted in relation to screening are applicable to other types of service.

## DEFINITIONS

Screening can be defined as the detection of a specific disease or a predisposing condition in people who are apparently healthy. *Mass* screening, sometimes termed *population* or *unselective* screening, involves screening an entire population in which there is no prior evidence of the presence of the condition in the individual. *Targetted* or *selective* screening is directed at sub-groups within the population where the risk is known to be concentrated. In the case of either mass screening or targetted screening the screening programme may be directed towards the detection of a single disease (*monophasic screening*) or there may be a battery of tests to look for a number of conditions in one individual (*multiphasic screeening*) (Hart 1992).

In recent years, the term 'screening' has come to include not only the identification of asymptomatic disease but also the identification of risk factors for disease, such as raised blood pressure, as well as unhealthy behaviours, such as smoking. These latter activities are more usually described as 'health promotion' which lies outside the province of screening, but in the context of today's pattern of major diseases some have argued that the distinction between screening and health promotion is becoming increasingly less useful (Holland & Stewart 1990).

## SCREENING CRITERIA

Several commentators, both in Britain and the USA, have drawn up criteria to be met in implementing screening programmes. Early criteria were elaborated in Britain by Wilson in the mid 1960s (Wilson & Junger 1968) and various modifications have since been elaborated (Cuckle & Wald 1984, Hudson et al 1988). Such criteria are not intended as blueprints for action. Their value lies in their drawing attention to the kinds of factors which purchasers, such as District Health Authorities, must consider when deciding whether or not to implement a screening programme, and which both purchasers and providers must take into account in evaluating screening programmes.

The most important criteria are grouped together in Box 8.1 under four headings: the disease, the test, follow-up and treatment, and economic costs (see also Ch. 10).

## DISCUSSION OF CRITERIA

### The disease

Most commentators stress that the disease being screened for must be

**Box 8.1** Screening criteria

*The disease*

The disease must be an important problem having a definite effect on length or quality of life.

It must have a recognized latent or early symptomatic stage, and the progression from this stage to the later symptomatic stage must be well understood.

*The test*

The diagnostic test must be reasonably accurate. A large proportion of 'false alarms' or a high rate of failure to detect the condition could be dangerously misleading.

The test must be acceptable to the population being screened, as well as to health care providers.

The test must be safe and simple to administer.

*Follow-up and treatment*

Screening must be a continuous process. Recall procedures must be effective.

When the initial test result is equivocal, further investigation should be undertaken quickly.

Test results should be communicated quickly and humanely to every individual tested.

There must be an effective treatment which improves the prognosis once a positive screening test result has been obtained.

Early intervention must be more effective that late intervention.

Resources and facilities must be available for follow-up diagnosis or treatment if required.

Follow-up interventions must be acceptable to patients and health care providers.

*Economic costs*

The cost of contacting the population, carrying out the tests, and subsequent treatments must be reasonable.

Costs must be economically balanced in relation to possible expenditure on medical care as a whole.

'important' but what counts as important is open to debate. Some suggest that the condition must be common while other suggest that it is justified to screen for a rare illness such as congenital hypothyroidism on the grounds of its seriousness and the effectiveness of treatment for this condition (Farmer & Miller 1991). Some suggest that trivial, non-life-threatening conditions should not be screened for while others point out that even trivial conditions, such as a build up of wax in the ear and resultant deafness, can have significant effects on the quality of life. In reality, when accurate tests and effective treatments exist, there are very few conditions which would not pass the criterion that they are 'important'. However, in attempting to determine priorities, purchasers might view relatively trivial and rare conditions as less important that common and serious problems.

The natural history of the disease is important in order to identify at what point the disease is detectable by screening and when intervention is likely to be effective. It is important that intervention is not too late (Farmer & Miller 1991). For example, it is known that the natural history of breast cancer is not the same for all women; the illness progresses at different speeds, particularly in different age groups. This is of crucial importance in considering the time interval between screens. If the interval between the early appearance of symptoms and the development of more advanced disease is much shorter than the interval between screens, then much disease in its earliest stages will be missed (Holland & Stewart 1990).

## The test

It is important that screening tests be reliable and valid. Conventionally, screening tests are measured in terms of their *sensitivity*, *specificity* and *predictive value*.

*Sensitivity* refers to the ability of the test to give a positive finding when the person being tested has the condition. The more sensitive the test, the greater the probability that the test result will be positive when the condition is present.

*Specificity* refers to the ability of the test to give a negative finding when the person being tested does not have the condition. The more specific the test, the greater the probability that the test result will be negative when the condition is absent. Thus, for any screening test there may be *false positives*, that is, 'false alarms' where the individual does not actually have the condition being sought by the test but has been falsely identified as positive. In addition, there may be *false negatives*, that is, people who do have the condition which the test has failed to detect (Hart 1992).

The more specific a test is, the less sensitive it is, and vice-versa. Hence trade-offs must be made between the two. High sensitivity is of paramount importance in order that as few people as possible slip through the net of detection. However, a highly sensitive test may limit specificity and give rise to a relatively high number of false positives. For some conditions, false positives greatly outnumber true positives.

*Predictive value* refers to the proportion of positive screening results that are correct. Predictive value is held to be the most important characteristic for any screening test (Mant & Fowler 1990, Holland & Stewart 1990). Where the predictive value of a screening programme is low, the costs, financial and other, of further investigating false positive results can be high. However, where the predictive value is too high, there is the danger of failing to detect an unacceptable number of those with the condition (Holland & Stewart 1990). Predictive value is related prevalence. Where prevalence is high, a positive test result is more likely to be a true positive; and where prevalence is low a positive result is more likely to be a false positive.

## Treatment and follow-up

All commentators stress that testing is of no benefit to the patient if no effective treatment exists for the condition being screened for. However, it should be pointed out that not all screening tests fulfil this criterion. For example, in recent years screening tests have been carried out for Huntington's disease, a genetically-determined illness for which there exists no effective treatment. In this instance, the possible benefits to patient of knowing 'one way or the other' are felt to justify screening in the absence of any effective treatment. This is a highly contentious area where the ethics of testing for a condition for which there are no effective treatments have been called into question by some.

It is generally agreed that screening should not be undertaken if equally effective treatment can be given once symptoms appear. For example, tuberculosis can now safely be left to the symptomatic stage before treatment is started, and hence Mass Miniature Radiography, carried out until the 1960s(?) has been withdrawn (Cochrane 1972). The comparative rarity of cases of TB in the whole population by the mid-1960s meant that 'unnecessary' presymptomatic detection was costing over £600 per case detected in 1966 (Cochrane 1972).

## Economic costs

What is a 'reasonable' cost depends in part on the seriousness of the condition. Detection of a treatable cancer would justify larger expenditure than detection of a trivial abnormality. The cost per case detected will depend on the prevalence of the condition, and its rate of progression. For example, radiological screening for lung cancer, which progresses quickly, would need to be repeated at least six monthly to be effective. This would be uneconomic. By contrast screening for asymptomatic bacteriuria once during pregnancy will pick up most cases, so this is justified in economic and medical terms (Teeling Smith 1975).

The use of resources to fund a screening programme denies those resources to other kinds of health care services. Thus, in deciding whether or not to provide a screening programme, the *opportunity costs* of so doing should always be carefully considered (see Ch. 7). For example, it might be decided that a screening programme is not the most beneficial use of resources and that resources devoted to screening could be deployed to greater effect elsewhere. Thus, the possibility that expenditure on other types of service than the screening programme being considered may result in greater net benefit to society as a whole must always be taken into account.

## THE COSTS AND BENEFITS OF SCREENING

As with any type of health service intervention, evaluation of screening programmes involves weighing up costs and benefits. Costs and benefits might be economic but they might also be personal or social.

In the following two sections we examine first the economists' approach to evaluating screening programmes. Drawing on the work of Paton (1992) we examine what is involved in thinking systematically about the costs and benefits of screening from an economic perspective. We then look at the ethics of screening and at some of the personal and social costs of screening.

## THE ECONOMICS OF SCREENING

In relation to screening, economists employ the same tools of analysis applicable across a wide range of activity. As we saw in Chapter 7, all techniques of economic evaluation measure costs. The measurement of costs is thus vital to purchasers, such as District Health Authorities, as a first stage in deciding on the costs and benefits of various screening programmes. In relation to cervical screening, Paton (1992) has suggested that costs might include:

1. the cost of the test, which includes both staff and equipment;
2. the costs of analysing the test results;
3. the cost of administering a call and recall service;
4. the costs of further diagnostic tests and treatment resulting from a positive test result;
5. costs incurred by patients, including time and travel.

In calculating costs, it is important to take into account the costs of follow-up treatment. A screening test for which there are inadequate follow-up services is neither ethical nor likely to be effective, and there is thus little value in calculations which exclude the costs of follow-up treatment.

Even where the costs of follow-up treatment are included, studies which look only at costs are of limited value since they do not relate costs to any outcome achieved. An expensive programme might be justified if the outcome was a significant reduction in mortality, but even a cheap programme could not be justified if it resulted in very few beneficial outcomes.

## Cost-effectiveness analysis

Cost-effectiveness studies are more helpful than a simple calculation of costs because costs are related to outcomes or benefits. We saw in Chapter 7 that cost-effectiveness studies can be used to compare alternative means of achieving the same objective. Hence if a Health Authority has already decided to implement a particular programme, for example, a programme of screening for cervical cancer, then it might wish to know the most cost-effective method of achieving its objective of reducing mortality from cervical cancer. Thus, a study of the cost-effectiveness of cervical screening might compare the cost-effectiveness of two methods, mass screening and targetted (selective) screening.

### A cost-effectiveness study of cervical screening (adapted from Paton 1992)

1. Define objective: to compare costs with 'life-years gained'.
2. State alternatives: mass screening versus targetted screening.
3. Determine costs: all costs associated with each alternative (see point 2 above).
4. Determine the number of life-years gained in relation to costs for each alternative.
5. Decide between alternatives.

## Cost–benefit analysis

Studies of cost-effectiveness are very useful in choosing between alternative means of dealing with the same problem, but they cannot aid decisions about how to choose between rival activities where the desired outcomes may differ. *Cost–benefit* analysis is broader in scope than cost-effectiveness analysis. It attempts to compare in monetary terms the total costs and total benefits of two or more competing activities, as an aid to purchasers' decisions about how to spend resources. For example the costs and benefits of carrying out coronary by-pass surgery could be compared with the costs and benefits of screening for coronary heart disease risk factors. The role of economists here is in describing and clarifying costs and benefits, but economic principles alone cannot 'decide' between competing activities (Paton 1992).

### Cost–benefit analysis (adapted from Paton 1992)

Define all costs and benefits of each alternative.
Quantify all costs and benefits in monetary terms.
Value benefits of each alternative.

## Screening versus not screening

We saw in Chapter 7 that the role of the economist is to aid decisions about whether to pursue one course of action or another. This might involve choosing between alternative interventions, or it might involve a choice between intervention and non-intervention. Below we illustrate the kinds of consideration which Health Authorities need to take into account when deciding whether or not to implement a particular screening programme (adapted from Paton 1992).

## Costs and benefits of screening

Costs of screening:

Costs of testing
Cost of treatment
Indirect cost of reducing mortality, e.g. pension payments to those whose premature death has been averted
Costs to patients in time
The cost of inducing anxiety in some patients

Benefits of screening:

Reduced premature mortality
Gain in productive capacity
Reassurance to patients
Saved cost of treatment at the symptomatic stage

## Costs and benefits of not screening

Costs of not screening:

Cost of treatment at the symptomatic stage
Premature mortality
Loss of productive capacity
Patients' fear of illness

Benefits of not screening:

Saved costs of testing and resultant treatment
Saved costs of reducing mortality, e.g. pension payments
Keeping patients in 'blissful ignorance'?

# The opportunity costs of screening

We saw in Chapter 7 that a consideration of opportunity costs is central to economics. Opportunity cost is the alternative benefits to be derived from a given resource. Spending resources on screening programmes is merely one use of available resources. The same resources could be put to other uses – either to funding other screening programmes, or to funding the treatment services which screening programmes need, or to funding an entirely different programme (Paton 1992).

In relation to screening, the dilemmas involved in determining opportunity costs are most acute where screening programmes compete for funds with the treatment services which the screening programme needs (Burke 1992, Paton 1992). For example, if no extra resources are made available for the detection and treatment of breast cancer, then the opportunity cost of devoting resources to improving breast cancer screening services is the lost opportunity to fund research into more effective treatments for the disease. Roberts (who died herself from breast cancer) has questioned whether screening for breast cancer is the best way of benefiting women. She has argued that screening is always a second best, an admission of the failure of prevention or treatment (Roberts et al 1985). In the wake of the recently implemented national programme of breast cancer screening a number of commentators have suggested that perhaps resources currently devoted to screening for breast cancer would be better used for research into more effective treatments. Clearly, for any type of screening programme, it is ethically indefensible to provide a screening programme where a failure to research the most effective treatment has resulted in second-rate treatments, or where follow-up treatment services are underfunded and unable to cope with a backlog of anxious patients (Holland & Stewart 1990, Burke 1992).

## THE ETHICS OF SCREENING

Weighing up the costs and benefits of screening involves important ethical considerations. These are discussed below.

### The efficacy of screening

An important difference between screening and other types of health service is that in the case of screening the health care professional is 'advertising' a service and promising a result (Cochrane 1972). The health care professional initiates the process, and implicit in the invitation to attend for screening is the assurance of help to the patient. The ethics of screening, therefore, are closely related to the question of whether the screening test achieves what the health care professional is claiming for it. To offer a screening test that does not meet basic criterion of efficacy, or to offer a test where there are no facilities for follow up are to make a contract that cannot be honoured (Burke 1992).

## INDIVIDUAL COSTS AND BENEFITS OF SCREENING

### Benefits

Of central importance is whether screening is beneficial. The principal benefit claimed for screening is that it prolongs the life of an individual in whom a treatable condition has been detected. This claim can be quantified. For example, in 1985 the yield of cervical cytology, in terms of lives saved, was estimated at 1 per 40 000 smear tests (Lancet 1985, Burke 1992). It is such evidence of the benefits of screening that gives rise to the view that to fail to screen for treatable conditions is ethically indefensible (Hart 1987, Burke 1992).

A second benefit claimed for screening is that early treatment may be less radical than later treatment and may cure some early cases (Chamberlain 1984, Holland & Stewart 1990).

Third, benefits can be reaped not only by those whose test results are positive. Negative results are said to provide reassurance (Chamberlain 1984, Grimes 1988). The counter-argument, however, is that prior to screening patients are unaware of many of the conditions they are screened for. It is the very act of screening them in the first place which gives rise to anxiety and a need for reassurance (Burke 1992).

## Costs

Against the above benefits must be weighed a number of potentially harmful consequences to the individual of screening.

First, the screening test itself may be hazardous (Chamberlain 1984). Some tests, such as mammography, carry risks. While the risks may be small at an individual level, the larger the number of tests, the greater the risk (Burke 1992).

Second, undergoing the test may have adverse psychological consequences, even where no abnormalities are detected. The very act of being tested may induce worry and introspection (Skrabanek 1988, Stoate 1989, Holland & Stewart 1990, Burke 1992).

Third, a positive test result, whether true or false, results in considerable psychological cost to the patient. Where the result is a true positive and effective treatment is available, the psychological cost of a positive test result may be acceptable to the patient. However, where no effective treatment exists and early diagnosis simply prolongs the period of time during which the condition is known about, the psychological burden of a positive test result may be unacceptable to the patient (Burke 1992). This is the dilemma in testing for such conditions as Huntington's disease.

Fourth, treatment following a positive test result may be harmful, that is, the cure may be worse than the disease. Screening increases the potential for harm arising from treatments that are unproven (Sackett & Holland 1975, Burke 1992).

Fifth, no test is completely sensitive and specific. A false-positive result will lead at least to a period of uncertainty and distress while further investigations are awaited, and at worst the individual will undergo unnecessary treatments (Holland & Stewart 1990). A false-negative is always very serious because it represents a failure on the part of the health professional to honour the contract to find and treat the patient's disorder, which is implicit in the invitation to attend for screening (Burke 1992).

Sixth, a false sense of security may arise also from patients' misinterpreting test results. A negative result such as normal blood pressure or a normal cholesterol level may be construed by individuals as justification for continuing their unhealthy life-style (Burke 1992). It has been suggested that screening creates a 'safety net' philosophy of reliance on health professionals to identify and solve health problems which saps individuals of a sense of self-responsibility for their own health (Holland & Stewart 1990).

Finally, there are some instances where screening may result in benefit to other members of society, but not necessarily to the person who is screened. An example is screening for the HIV virus. While other members of society may benefit from an individual's identification as HIV positive, the individual may or may not benefit. Certainly there are costs to the individual – the cost of knowing that s/he has an incurable illness, and the stigmatization that may result from others' knowledge of his/her HIV positive status (Burke 1992).

## SCREENING AND INEQUALITIES IN HEALTH

### Screening and the 'inverse care law'

In 1971 Julian Tudor Hart formulated his 'inverse care law' which referred to the fact that those people most in need of medical care are the least likely to receive it (Hart 1971; see also Ch. 5). There is some evidence that Hart's 'law' applies also to many screening programmes. In order to achieve the outcomes of reducing mortality or morbidity, screening programmes require a high uptake rate, particularly amongst vulnerable groups (Coulter & Baldwin 1987, Farmer &

Miller 1991). As we saw in Chapters 5 and 7, both access to, and uptake of, services tend to be poorer among those in the lower social classes. For example, the rate of uptake of cervical screening is lower in social classes IV and V than in higher social groups (Farmer & Miller 1991). Many screening programmes have problems of coverage, with low-risk individuals attending screening programmes and high-risk individuals staying away. In some cases, coverage has not been sufficient to alter patterns of morbidity or mortality (Robson & Speigal 1992). Even where mortality and morbidity rates have improved for society as a whole, the improvement may be far less for those in social classes IV and V than for those in the higher social classes. Burke (1992) suggests that inequalities in uptake are a particular problem in the private sector where screening programmes have been initiated not by health care professionals but by consumer groups. Such programmes may fail to reach those most in need of screening. This is not to suggest, however, that the problem is confined to the private sector.

## SCREENING: A CASE STUDY OF CERVICAL CANCER

In the following case study we evaluate screening for cervical cancer against the criteria set out at the start of this chapter. Our case study draws heavily on Ridsdale (1992).

### The disease must be an important problem

Cervical cancer is an important problem. In 1984, 1899 women in England and Wales died of the disease, and 4043 new cases were diagnosed. The disease is both common and serious.

### The natural history and progression of the disease must be well understood

The causes of cervical cancer, and the way in which it progresses, are not well understood. However, it is recognized that there are stages in the development of the disease from mild, to moderate, to severe dysplasia. Severe dysplasia is recognized as an early stage of cervical cancer.

### Early intervention must be more effective than late intervention

One way to assess whether early intervention is more effective than late is to compare those populations who have offered comprehensive screening with those who have not. Differences in mortality will show the benefits of early identification and treatment. In Iceland, between 1965 and 1982 a nationwide programme of screening of all age groups resulted in a drop in mortality of 80%. In Finland, over the same period, screening was targeted at a smaller age range and was conducted less frequently. Here, the reduction in mortality was only 50%. In Norway, where only 5% of the population was covered by organized screening, mortality declined by only 10%. In Britain during the same period the decline in mortality was 21%. Such evidence suggests that screening and early intervention is more effective.

Another way of looking at whether early detection is more effective is to look at the screening status of women who have developed cancer. In a study of women who had died from cervical cancer, 90% had never been screened (Spriggs & Boddington 1976).

### The test must be reasonably accurate
Smear tests tend to underestimate the presence of disease. A single smear has a false-negative rate of about 40%.

### The test must be acceptable to the population being screened
Some women do not accept the invitation to attend for screening. There are a number of reasons for this. They might find the appointment time inconvenient; or they may not understand the reason for screening, and see it as unimportant. To some women the test is not acceptable because they are embarrassed about an internal examination. Some 60% of women prefer to see a female health professional for screening, but in 1987 over 10 000 GPs serving over 20 million patients had no woman partners (Standing & Mercer 1984, Ridsdale 1992). Women who belong to ethnic minorities, particularly Asian women, prefer the test to be carried out by a woman (McAvoy & Raza 1988). In many GP practices screening is undertaken by a female nurse. A survey of 300 practice nurses carried out by Greenfield et al in 1987 found that 70% were taking cervical smears. There is some evidence that screening programmes are more effective where practice nurses are involved than where GPs are working alone (Fullard et al 1987).

### Resources and facilities must be available for follow-up diagnosis or treatment if required
There can be hold-ups in follow-up interventions from GPs surgeries,

from patients finding telephone lines engaged, to waiting lists for colposcopy clinics, to waiting lists for hospital admission. The extent to which follow-up facilities are deemed adequate depends on clinical opinion about the appropriate stage at which to refer on women with abnormalities. There is agreement that severe dysplasia requires referral, but less agreement about the best way to proceed with women whose smears reveal only mild or moderate dysplasia. If all women with moderate dysplasia were referred, there would be further bottlenecks in the system. There are variations in practice throughout the country to deal with moderate dysplasia. Some women are asked to return for a repeat smear test in a given period, others may be referred for colposcopy straight away. If all women in Britain with mild dyskaryosis were referred for colposcopy, current NHS treatment facilities would not be adequate.

## Screening must be a continuous process

Screening must be performed at sufficiently frequent intervals to detect abnormalities before the appearance of overt disease. Data from Europe and North America suggest that if all women were screened at least once before the age of 35, and were then re-screened at 5-year intervals, there would be a reduction of 84% in the cumulative incidence of cancer. Screening at 3-year intervals would reduce the cumulative incidence by 91%. There are difficult questions concerning the optimal screening interval for women where moderate dyskaryosis has been detected. It has been argued that if colposcopy services were freely available, that all such women would benefit from the service, rather than re-screening (Fox 1987). The screening interval for those with mild dyskaryosis is also a controversial subject. Follow-up of these women shows that up to 26% will progress to the severe stage in 2 years, but half can revert to normal (Campion et al 1986, Robertson et al 1988). In the light of the high frequency of this abnormality, the differences in outcome, and the scarcity of resources, recommendations vary from colposcopy to a repeat smear in 6 months to 1 year.

## Costs must be economically balanced in relation to possible expenditure on medical care as a whole

There have been few studies of the economic costs and benefits of cervical screening. However, it has been estimated by Ridsdale (1992) that in the mid 1980s, approximately £20 million was spent in an attempt to prevent 1785 deaths in the over-35s, and £25 million in an attempt to prevent 114 deaths in the under-35s. Because of the high cost-to-benefit ratio, it has been argued that the same investment would prevent more deaths in other areas of the NHS (Roberts et al 1985). However, the high cost per life saved reflects the fact that those with a lower risk (the under-35s) were screened more frequently. As with any screening programme, the additional benefits per cost of each screening test decrease as the programme is extended to those at lower risk. It has been suggested that 5-yearly testing of women aged over 35 is the most cost-effective option.

## CONCLUSION

In this chapter we have illustrated the way in which principles and methods derived from a range of disciplines and perspectives – epidemiology, sociology, economics and ethics – can be applied in evaluating one particular type of health service, screening. This chapter concludes our discussion of the various theoretical and ethical perspectives which can be brought to bear on health needs assessment. In the following three chapters we discuss some of the more practical aspects of health needs assessment.

# A framework for local health needs assessment

# 9

## LOCAL HEALTH NEEDS ASSESSMENT IN PRACTICE

Until now, *Health Needs Assessment* has been mainly concerned with diverse theoretical perspectives and the competing tensions and arguments between them when needs assessment activities are proposed. While an understanding of these various positions is essential to the intelligent appreciation of what is possible in health needs assessment, it can leave practitioners feeling that there is no way forward. Hence we return in Chapters 9 to 11 to the theme of practical, local, health needs assessment. This is not to deny the relevance of what has gone before, but to recognise that practitioners in the field have to *act*, albeit in the knowledge that their actions will always be susceptible to criticism from one theoretical perspective or another. In this chapter therefore we explore the central elements which appear to some extent in all local, practical, health needs assessments. If it is possible to describe a 'framework' for local health needs assessment then it can be said to encompass the following criteria:

population definition and selection;
problem definition and measurement;
comprehensiveness;
outcomes;
resources.

The issues which are described under the above headings are not neatly compartmentalized and frequently overlap. Different approaches also tend to place greater emphasis on some aspects of the assessment than on others. This reinforces the point that there is no *one* agreed way to carry out health needs assessment exercises. For examples we draw largely on work by four sets of authors in this field (Jenkins 1990, Stirland & Raftery 1992, Hawtin et al 1994, Pickin & St Leger 1994). It will be seen that their recommendations on what to include, how the material is presented, and the overall structure of health needs assessment, vary considerably. What they demonstrate, however, is some of the ways in which practitioners, sometimes with different professional orientations and objectives, have responded to the need to *act* in the face of so many competing theoretical perspectives on health needs assessment. In Chapter 10 we shall describe how one Director of Public Health (DPH) went about presenting an assessment of health needs of the people of Nottingham in her annual reports to the health authority and in Chapter 11 how health visitors and undergraduate nurses have carried out local health profiling exercises.

## POPULATION DEFINITION AND SELECTION

### Administrative boundaries

All health needs assessment takes place within a geographical locality. This might vary from an entire nation (see Chapter 4 on the *Health of the Nation*), or it might be a very small area such as an electoral ward or civil parish. The 10-yearly (decennial) Census is a major source of baseline information on numerous population variables from country level down to the smallest aggregate unit of approximately 200 households known as an enumeration district. (*An Introductory Guide to the 1991 Census* (Leventhal et al 1993) and *The 1991 Census User's Guide* (Dale & Marsh 1993) are invaluable sources of information on the Census. In particular, Chapter 3 in Dale & Marsh (1993) on Census Geography gives a comprehensive review of the geographical areas used in the Census.) The choice of population clearly depends upon the specific purpose of the health needs assessment exercise. In some instances the choice is pre-determined. For example, District Health Authorities (DHAs) and local authorities are required to study all those who reside within their particular administrative (geographical) areas. These are particularly useful for comparative purposes as these administrative areas usually coincide with those used in many government publications (e.g. the Census and employment data). These publications provide valuable information on health-influencing factors such as employment, housing and social class which can be used to deduce the life circumstances of the population whose health needs are being assessed (see Ch. 6 on Epidemiological approaches to health needs assessment, and Ch. 5 on Inequalities in health and health care). Many health authorities undertake locality-based needs assessment in which the needs of people living in different geographical localities within the wider population of a City or County are assessed. These are used as a basis for decisions about targetting resources towards particular localities (Pickin & St Leger 1994). For example, the health needs of people living in relatively affluent localities might be assessed and compared with those people living in more deprived areas. Two of the sets of authors referred to later in this chapter are concerned with health needs assessment for people with mental health problems or learning disabilities (Jenkins 1990, Stirland & Raftery 1992).

A number of other health needs assessment exercises are also based on administrative but non-geographical considerations. For example, a health needs assessment exercise initiated within a general practice may cover all the patients on that practice's list. Similarly, health needs assessment carried out by a health visitor may cover all those clients on her case load. There are problems however with using such populations for comparative purposes in the way that health authorities use locality-based assessments. Because they overlap several administrative boundaries (such as wards, parishes or even DHA boundaries) it is not possible to know the characteristics of the *total population* from which a practice list or health visitor's case load is drawn. If, for example, a general practitioner's (GP's) practice list appears to contain a disproportionately large number of elderly people, it is usually not possible (because the list does not relate to one specific geographical area) to identify *accurately* how representative it is of the larger population from which it is drawn.

In carrying out health needs assessment it is important to reflect on whether *knowing* the extent of a population's representativeness compared to other populations *matters* for the purposes for which an assessment is intended. If the assessment is to be used to argue for a re-distribution of resources in order to achieve greater equity in the provision of services between a poor and an affluent area, then reliable comparisons are essential. On the other hand, if the assessment is to identify the extent of some need within a specific population in order to set objectives for service provision (such as, say, establishing a diabetic clinic for elderly people within a GP's surgery, see Ch. 11) then it is essential to know the extent of the problem within the GP's list, but it is of less interest (at least to the GP and practice staff) to compare the distribution of elderly diabetics on their list with that occurring in the wider population from which it is drawn.

The choice of a study population in health needs assessment is therefore dependent on the purposes for which it is intended, for there are a number of different ways of looking at the needs of the sub-groups within it. In Chapter 6 on epidemiological approaches to health needs assessment, the ways in which the characteristics of baseline (or denominator) information are used as a basis for comparison with the characteristics of the population being studied, were considered.

## PROBLEM DEFINITION AND MEASUREMENT

### Community needs assessment

In Chapter 1 the fact that health needs assessment activities are carried out by a wide variety of people from varying backgrounds was discussed. Local needs assessment may be carried out either by health care professionals or by voluntary or community groups as a means of documenting the extent of unmet needs in their community. Hawtin et al (1994) discuss what is meant by a community. One conception of community is that of a group of people who live or work in the same geographical area. However, communities can also be defined in terms of an administrative area such as a school catchment area, or an area served by a particular health authority. A third way of thinking about community is as a group of people with a shared interest arising out of shared characteristics. For example, women, ethnic minorities, children and people with disabilities might be viewed as communities of interest. However, there can be difficulties with this approach. For example, it might not be helpful to focus on the 'black community'. Although all black people might have a shared interest in overcoming white racism, the idea of a 'black community' might be insensitive to the many differences between different peoples. Hawtin et al (1994) stress that this is not an argument against focusing on particular groups; rather, they urge, we should remain aware of the many differences within communities.

There are many different kinds of problem which a DHA might attempt to address. One type of problem is to identify the needs of a particular client group such as the elderly, disabled people, the mentally ill, children and people with learning difficulties. Second, it is possible to focus on specific diseases, such as heart disease, diabetes or cancer. Third, some forms of health needs assessment focus on particular interest groups, that is, groups of people with a shared interest arising out of shared characteristics, such as the black community, or the Jewish community or the gay community. Fourth, it is possible to focus on particular services, such as screening services. Finally, it is possible to look at a particular factor which is known to affect health, such as unemployment or housing. In Chapter 10 on health profiling at the DHA level it will be seen that most of these aspects of health needs assessment have been covered at some time in one health authority.

## Demographic characteristics

Pickin & St Leger (1994) take as their starting point for assessing health needs the fact that *age* and *gender* are the main determinants of both health and the use of health services in any population. They divide the population into nine age groups from before birth to old age. After age 15, each age group is also divided by gender. The division of the population into age groups, and their further subdivision by sex, is both a practical way of dividing up the population to be studied, and also expresses their theoretical position that the most powerful influences on health are related to age and sex.

Pickin & St Leger therefore adopt a strongly *epidemiological* approach to health needs assessment. Having divided the population by age and sex, they then adopt the same basic approach to assessing needs within each group. Within each age group they look at the following factors (Pickin & St Leger 1994):

- the main influences on health and the leading causes of mortality and morbidity;
- sources of information relating to morbidity, mortality and demography (population structure);

- the ways in which people's health experience may be modified by socio-economic, environmental, ethnic and cultural factors (modifiers);
- health resources – these include resources within the individual, family and community, as well as formal services delivered by health services, local authorities, and the voluntary and private sectors;
- the way in which people's access to, and use of, services is modified by socio-economic, environmental, ethnic and cultural factors (modifiers);
- primary care services which are currently available to people in each age group, as well as possible new services.

## Multi-dimensional perspectives on problem assessment

Stirland & Raftery (1992) suggest that there are four dimensions of 'need' which should to be taken into account in mental health needs assessment. These are:

- the *amount* of mortality, and the *amount* and *nature* of morbidity arising from mental disorder;
- the *demand* for care;
- the *wishes and aspirations* of patients and their carers and other local residents and the *views* of professionals in the primary and secondary health care sectors;
- the capacity of the individual to benefit from treatment and support.

Thus, needs are not defined by Stirland and Raftery simply as health problems. Need is also defined as the 'capacity to benefit from health care'. Moreover, in defining needs, the demands, views and aspirations of those other than health care professionals must be taken into account. Stirland & Raftery (1992) suggest that their model of health needs assessment raises some basic questions:

- how much mental illness is there? Who suffers from mental ill-health? What kinds of mental health problems do people suffer from?
- what services are provided? Who is using them? Are they accessible? How are they organized?
- what services are needed to prevent, treat or rehabilitate people

with mental disorders? What are the expected benefits from these services?

- what are patients' and carers' priorities? How satisfied are they with the services they currently receive?
- how much is being spent on health care for mental illness. Is this good value for money or are there more cost-effective and acceptable alternatives?

Stirland and Raftery acknowledge that much of the information needed to answer these questions is lacking. They contend, however, that such questions are helpful in providing a framework within which such information as exists can be used in a meaningful and appropriate way, and in drawing attention to the areas in which knowledge is lacking.

Stirland and Raftery begin by looking at some of the demographic and socio-economic characteristics of the population resident within the administrative district where they based their assessment (Wandsworth DHA). However, they choose particularly those characteristics which are likely to affect both people's risk of experiencing mental health problems, and their use of services. (These are equivalent to Pickin and St Leger's 'modifiers'.) It can be seen that they include many *social* indicators. They look, for example at the age and sex structure of the District; at the proportion of Afro-Caribbean and Asian people; the number of single-person households; single-parent families; and pensioners living alone or with an elderly partner. They note too the growing numbers of homeless people. Using the Jarman index of social deprivation, Stirland and Raftery are able to ascertain that Wandsworth is a socially deprived district, although there is great variation between the various electoral wards within the District of Wandsworth. (The Jarman index was discussed in Ch. 3.)

## Goal setting as a means of prioritizing problems

A different approach is adopted by Jenkins (1990). She takes a *client group* approach in developing a model for health needs assessment for mental health care. However, she appears to be *less* concerned with population mental health needs assessment than with the health authorities' *objectives* for mental health services. As we have seen, many approaches to health needs assessment suggest that the first task is to identify needs; the second to review all the available resources, and only finally to identify what goals or outcomes we are trying to achieve. Jenkins, in discussing the role of health authorities in assessing mental health care needs, suggests that it is best *first* to formulate objectives or goals. Her approach is therefore very much in line with the *Health of the Nation* strategy for target setting (NHS Management Executive 1993c). Jenkins argues that at a time of comparatively easy access to large quantities of data, it is vital to think critically about how we intend to use such data, and not to let the data dictate the questions we can answer. She suggests that the most fruitful approach which health authorities can take is to begin by setting objectives (targets); secondly, to choose appropriate strategies; and only finally to use existing data to determine whether these strategies are being implemented and how well the objectives are being achieved.

Jenkins sets out a possible approach to assessing, evaluating and monitoring over time the health needs of people with a range of mental disorders and disabilities. She adopts the same approach in relation to a range of conditions from schizophrenia and dementia to learning disabilities (Jenkins uses the term 'mental handicap'). For example, in the case of mental handicap, Jenkins begins by reviewing what is known in terms of prevalence and incidence; pre-disposition to mental and physical illnesses; longevity; and the estimated need for educational, health and care facilities. She then asks preliminary basic questions concerning the scope for improvements on a range of fronts:

- can incidence be reduced?
- can relapse and readmission rates be reduced?
- is there an avoidable mortality?

She then formulates a number of possible objectives centred around what might be achievable, and suggests indicators which would tell us about whether strategies for achieving the objectives were being implemented. Following Donabedian (1980), Jenkins classifies the data conventionally used by health authorities to assess health needs into input, process and outcome indicators. Inputs measure what resources and services are available such as finance, personnel, hospital buildings and services such as inpatient and outpatient facilities. Inputs might include the following facilities:

- an ante-natal screening service for genetic disorders;
- an acute admission ward for the mentally ill together with agreed staffing levels;

- a respite service for the long term mentally ill.

Processes are concerned with how care is organised and carried out. They are about the activities undertaken in the health care system and might include:

- what proportion of ante-natal mothers were screened for which genetic disorders, and with what results?
- how many people were admitted during a year to an acute admission ward, and with what mental disorders?
- how many people used a respite service during a year?

Outcomes are about the end results. They are about changes in people's health and are frequently limited to mortality and morbidity rates. However, Jenkins suggests the following indicators in the context of health services for those with mental handicap:

- a reduction in the incidence of mental handicap;
- prevention of additional disability and premature mortality;
- equity of access to health services for the mentally handicapped compared with the general population;
- improved self-esteem and reduced psychiatric morbidity;
- care for the carers.

## COMPREHENSIVENESS

Almost any kind of health needs assessment breaks up the totality of people's experience. 'Health problems' and 'social problems' are often studied separately (although as has been seen throughout *Health Needs Assessment*, the two are frequently intimately related). While it is not always a practical proposition that health needs assessment exercises should cover every kind of difficulty in all areas of people's lives, it is important not to lose sight of the fact that people's experiences cannot be neatly compartmentalized (Hawtin et al 1994). This was the point made in the quotation from Frankenberg (1969) in the Foreword. As an anthropologist studying a community, he was frustrated by his inability to obtain a sense of the inter-connectedness of people's lives. Similar difficulties are experienced by practitioners carrying out local health needs assessment exercises. In practical terms this means that the various agencies and groups who assess needs must collaborate, and be aware of the relationship between problems which are conventionally designated as 'health problems' and those designated as 'social problems'. Thus, for example, although health authorities are charged with assessing health needs, and local authorities with the need for social care, the two kinds of need are frequently inter-related, so that health authorities and local authorities profit greatly when they collaborate closely (Hawtin et al 1994). Similarly, health care practitioners in day-to-day contact with clients cannot ignore the totality of their clients' life experiences and problems. An assessment of the needs, for example, of a patient with cancer should ideally be concerned with not only the patients' health needs but also with her entire 'neediness', which may include not only health needs but also social, economic and spiritual needs.

True to their pro-active community orientation, Hawtin et al (1994, pp. 5–13) include comprehensiveness in their definition of a community profile:

> A comprehensive description of the needs of a population that is defined, or defines itself, as a community, and the resources that exist within that community, carried out with the active involvement of the community itself, for the purpose of developing an action plan or other means of improving the quality of life in the community.

Like other models of health needs assessment, the focus of Hawtin et al is not only on needs but also on resources, and on the outcome of 'improving the quality of life' of the community. In this definition, profiling should be *comprehensive*, it should focus on the *needs* and *resources* of the *community*, it should draw on the *active involvement* of the community, and it must result in a plan of *action*. For this reason, Hawtin et al argue that, although many community profiles are not comprehensive, they should be. They argue that although much is known, for example about the relationship between poor housing and ill health, in practice policy has often failed to act on this knowledge. Hawtin et al argue that community profiles which are comprehensive can challenge existing 'bureaucratic departmentalism' by their more accurate reflection of the reality of people's lives.

## OUTCOMES

Most commentators agree that an important objective or outcome of health needs assessment is to bring about 'health gain'. Clearly, the particular health gain sought depends in part on what need is being assessed. In many types of health need assessment the desired type of health gain is a reduction in mortality. However, this is not always an appropriate or achievable objective. A reduction in morbidity is another common outcome towards which health needs assessment might aspire. Outcomes or objectives can include not only those which 'add years to life', but also those which add 'life to years'. Improving 'quality of life' is therefore also another important outcome. Other types of outcome contain the objective of promoting equity between different sections of society. This outcome is often expressed in the objective of improving the access of disadvantaged groups to essential services. Finally, some outcomes relate not to those people whose health problems are being assessed but to their carers. Providing support to carers is thus another important objective of health needs assessment.

The measurement of *outcome* is probably the most complex task. This is because health outcomes, such as changes in morbidity and mortality are the result not only of health care interventions but also of wider social changes and policies which affect health, such as policies concerned with the environment or general changes in living standards. Health service administrators and health authorities have frequently used measures of processes as proxy measures for outcomes because data on outcomes is both hard to obtain and difficult to interpret. For example, health authorities often measure how well a service is used on the assumption that the use of a particular service is equal to the success of that service in bringing about a beneficial health outcome. Of course such an assumption cannot be made. Input and process data do not really tell us about outcomes, but they are sometimes the only kind of data available.

For Stirland & Raftery (1992) 'health gain' is the outcome towards which health needs assessment is striving and they include 'the capacity of the individual to benefit from treatment and support' as one of four dimensions of need. In relation to mental health, health gains are defined by Stirland and Raftery as:

- reduction in avoidable mortality and morbidity;
- maintenance of an adequate level of social functioning;
- improved consumer experience.

Hawtin et al (1994) emphasize that a community profile should include a plan of action which sets goals and targets for improving the quality of life of members of the community, and Pickin & St Leger (1994) stress that one of the most important elements of health needs assessment is its concern with the question of what we are trying achieve. It is vital therefore to think about what outcomes we desire to bring about. They suggest four possible broad goals which those responsible for assessing health needs, such as DHAs, might pursue (Pickin & St Leger 1994):

Increasing population health overall;
The maximization of health potential;
A reduction in unacceptable variations in health;
Equity in the use of resources.

Pickin and St Leger thus suggest that it is important to pursue both *health gains* and *equity*. They argue that the above four broad goals need not be incompatible, although each places constraints on the others. Here is a pragmatic example of an attempt at compromise between different theoretical perspectives on health needs assessment. It has been seen in Chapter 7 (Economics, utilitarianism and health needs assessment) and Chapter 5 (Inequalities in health and health care) that, in practice, it is virtually impossible to reconcile the utilitarian objective of the maximization of health potential with the egalitarian objective of equity in the use of resources. This is why, at the end of the day, governments can only suggest compromise between the different positions. Indeed, in deciding on what health outcomes we desire, Pickin and St Leger acknowledge that value-judgements are important. They acknowledge that professional definitions of need may differ from lay definitions, and they suggest that a process is needed by which the local community's perspective can be included in decisions about health needs and the benefits of various interventions (Pickin & St Leger 1994). Although it would be hard to disagree with any of the above arguments for setting objectives for health needs assessment, they all lack the precision of Jenkins' (1990) approach to goal setting as a basis for health needs assessment. Her approach undoubtedly stands out in its emphasis on the need for a precise definition of outcomes as the basis for defining the health needs of a client group.

The general lack of precision in defining outcomes in health needs assessment reflects both the practical and political difficulties referred to in the introduction to this chapter. Outcomes research is an area where large amounts of research energy and resources are currently being directed, and hopefully much greater clarity may be expected in this area in future (Long 1994, Brettle et al 1995, French 1995). The idea of setting objectives in terms of targets as advocated by the *Health of the Nation* has not yet entered the literature on health needs assessment to any large extent. Undoubtedly this will change as DHAs become more experienced at working in these ways, although in Chapter 10 it will be suggested that DHAs are in a praradoxical position, being required as purchasers to assess the health needs of their population, but then only being able to influence outcomes at second hand through the providers from whom they purchase services. The difficulties should not be under-estimated for, as has been discussed, there is no consensus as to what is seen as a beneficial outcome from health care interventions.

## RESOURCES IN HEALTH NEEDS ASSESSMENT

Resources for health gain have already been mentioned at various points within the context of the frameworks which the four sets of authors advance for carrying out health needs assessment. Health resources are frequently equated with financial resources, and with formal health care services. However, Pickin & St Leger (1994) suggest that health resources are more widely distributed and that these need to be included within any health needs assessment. Many health resources exist within individuals themselves, within the family and within the local community. Health resources which are to be found within the formal services include not only health care services but also local authorities, the private sector and the voluntary sector.

Stirland and Raftery's model of health needs assessment, like that of Pickin and St Leger, links health problems or health needs to the resources available to address these needs appropriately and effectively, in pursuit of the outcome of bringing about health gains. Stirland and Raftery's approach is represented in the following model (Stirland & Raftery 1992, p. 128):

NEEDS......................RESOURCES......................HEALTH GAIN

Like Pickin and St Leger, Stirland and Raftery do not define resources in a narrow way. Resources include (Stirland & Raftery 1992):

- service facilities, including hospital beds, clinics, day centres, supported housing and sheltered occupation;

- the interventions available for prevention, treatment and care;
- the people and skills required to meet the various dimensions of 'need';
- expenditure on service provision.

Resources are also defined widely by Hawtin et al (1994) as the assets held by, and benefitting, the community. These include hospitals, housing stock, community centres and parks. They include people's time and expertise, a range of services, and employment opportunities. Hawtin et al point out that the resources currently available may be under-utilized, and that there may be potential resources, for example vacant land or derelict buildings which could in future be used. They stress too that some resources are less tangible than others. Many intangible resources, such as support networks among families, friends and neighbours can be a great source of strength. It is important to look at a community's strengths and not simply at its deficiencies. Finally, although financial resources are clearly important, Hawtin et al stress that extra money is not always the only way of meeting need.

## CONCLUSION

In this Chapter, five separate components of health needs assessment have been considered in the context of the different approaches adopted by authors who have addressed these issues in some depth. All health needs assessment concerns three central elements: health problems (need), resources, and outcomes (health gain). It has been seen throughout *Health Needs Assessment* that none of these elements is unproblematic. Even the authors cited in this chapter, who are pragmatic realists in their approach to health needs assessment, recommend that the task should be undertaken in different ways and give greater emphasis to one aspect rather than another. Despite the pragmatic approach, the ways in which needs and health gain (or outcomes) are viewed still depends very much on implicit underlying theoretical perspectives.

# Local health needs assessment: reports of the Director of Public Health

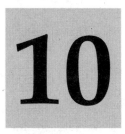

**10**

■ **CONTENTS**

## INTRODUCTION

The annual reports of the local Medical Officers of Health, dating back historically to the second half of the 18th century, have re-emerged in the 1990s in modern format following the Report of a Committee of Inquiry into the Future Development of the Public Health Function (Public Health in England 1988) and the NHS and Community Care Act (Department of Health 1990). Produced by the District Health Authority (DHA) offices of local Directors of Public Health, these periodic reports on the state of the health of the population within district health authorities are now concerned with health needs assessment as a basis for purchasing health care. In the reformed NHS, the role of purchasing DHAs is to assess the health needs of the populations they serve, and to monitor over time whether they are meeting the population's health needs. Health needs assessment requires that DHAs undertake an initial baseline assessment of the health of the population resident within the district's geographical boundaries, since this is viewed as an essential first step in monitoring and evaluating progress in meeting needs through the purchase of health services (Jenkins 1990). An assessment of the total burden of ill health is seen as necessary for judging the appropriateness of the services currently being delivered by providers and for determining priorities for the future. The rationale is that services must be matched to identified needs (Drummond 1993).

In undertaking this baseline assessment of health needs, DHAs rely on the epidemiological expertise of their Directors of Public Health (DPH). The DPH in each DHA produces an annual report of the health of its resident population. Its aims are to describe and interpret data concerning the health status of the resident population; to identify health problems and the extent to which they are being addressed; to evaluate existing services, and to make recommendations for the future. The DPH's report serves as a guide to those responsible for decisions about the allocation of resources for the purchase of services. Its recommendations form an important basis for such decisions (Jenkins 1990). In the discussion of local health needs assessment at DHA level which follows we are taking the annual reports of the DPH for Nottingham DHA as a case study of what has been achieved since 1990. This is not to say that the Nottingham reports are necessarily typical of all DHAs in their presentation. Extracts from them are used here for two purposes. First, to demonstrate how it is possible to keep in mind complex theoretical perspectives on health needs assessment whilst still needing to *act* in a pragmatic way. The five criteria of population and problem definition, comprehensiveness, resources and outcomes are all addressed throughout the reports and reference is made to the problems of defining need, resource and health gain, both separately and in relation to each other. Second, the reports are used as an illustration of how the rich sources of local information which are now available for every health district have been used for the purposes of local DHA health needs assessment.

## ASSESSMENT OF HEALTH NEEDS IN NOTTINGHAM

In 1990, Dr Lindsey Davies, DPH for Nottingham, wrote in the Preface of her first annual Report on the health of the people of Nottingham (Nottingham Health Authority 1990, p. 1): 'The assessment of health needs is a daunting task. In this first report, we have chosen to offer a broad overview of the population's health and to complement this by a more searching discussion of a small number of important local health issues'. This first report for Nottingham DHA as a purchasing authority referred to the great changes and challenges facing health authorities and local authorities as they prepared for changes in funding and operation as a result of the implementation of the NHS and Community Care Act, 1990. It referred to the requirement to assess health needs before entering into service agreements (an early form of purchasing arrangement) with hospitals and other service providers in order to ensure that the needs would be met. The 1990 report was cautious in scope and a commitment was made to address further topics in detail in later reports. This indeed happened, and in successive annual reports the following issues were addressed in detail:

- 1991, Health of the elderly, mental health, and the elderly mentally ill (Nottingham Health Authority 1991);
- 1992, Health of people with physical disabilities, cancer, smoking, and communicable disease (Nottingham Health Authority 1992);
- 1993, Healthy pregnancy, health in infancy, health in children, health of people with learning disabilities and accidents (Nottingham Health Authority 1993);
- 1995, Aiming for health in the year 2000 (Health and deprivation, Nottingham Health Authority 1995).

## Population and problem definition

Thus, Nottingham District Health Authority set out systematically to define and measure 'problems' relating to the health of the total population living within its administrative boundaries. As the DPH said in the quotation referred to above, the task was daunting and therefore the establishment of a baseline definition for all the population sub-groups involved was planned to take place over several years. It can also be seen that the definition of 'problems' is not homogenous as, in some cases, they involve the health of people with diseases entities such as cancer or communicable disease, in others they are concerned with demographic sub-groups (infancy and children), and in others with factors associated with lifestyles such as deprivation and smoking.

## Comprehensiveness

The need to be comprehensive in the assessment of health needs was recognised by the DPH in her initial discussion. She points out that no assessment of health need can avoid conceptual questions about the nature of 'health' and the nature of 'need'. She recognizes that health is a broad concept, captured only partially and inadequately in the available information on which her report must rely. Nottingham's DPH is acutely aware that the measures of health such as mortality and morbidity indicators do not fully capture the health status of the community (Nottingham Health Authority 1990). Moreover, she stresses that we should not lose sight of the broad idea that 'health' is not an end in itself but is a means of promoting social participation (Nottingham Health Authority 1990). This perspective is reminiscent of Doyal and Gough's view that health and autonomy are inter-related and that being healthy and autonomous about being able to function in a social world (see Ch. 2).

The distinction between need and demand is also of crucial practical importance to DHAs. In Chapter 2 it was seen that several authors consider that need is not a value-neutral concept, and that what counts as a health need is a contestable question. *Who* decides what is a health need is acknowledged by Nottingham's DPH as a crucial question. She recognizes that consumer-defined needs and expert-defined needs may come into conflict. The DPH's 1990 report is largely based on her own expert definition of need but she recognizes that hers is not the only perspective on need and that consumer perspectives must be taken into account. This is clearly an area where nurses have an important role to play as mediators between the public and DHA public health departments. Practising nurses are well placed to describe some of the needs of the population and to make this information available to public health departments.

## Demography

Demography is the starting point of the Nottingham DPH's 1990 report. Since illness and death are related to the age structure of the population, demographic projections are essential for health care planning. The DPH's (1990) report shows that in Nottingham the proportion of people over the age of 85 will roughly double by the year 2010 from about seven thousand to about fourteen and a half thousand. As this age group is the largest consumer of health and social residential services this statistic will clearly have an important bearing on services provided for elderly people in the future, especially if the figure is extrapolated to the country as a whole and it is recognized that *all* DHAs will be confronting a similar increase in demand.

## Assessing the total burden of mortality and morbidity: mortality

In order to obtain a picture of total mortality, the most useful source of information is the Standardized Mortality Ratio which is a way of expressing a local death rate so that it is directly comparable with other parts of the country, even though their population structure may be different. The Nottingham 1990 report found that mortality in Nottingham was the same as the average for England and Wales, however, when the information is broken down for different electoral wards great differences emerge.

Different causes of mortality are more likely in different age groups. There are also important differences between men and women. It is therefore helpful to break down total mortality rates into rates for each cause of death in both sexes. In her 1990 report, Nottingham's DPH examines the leading causes of death within each age group as well as variations between the sexes.

In the age group from 1 month to 14 years there were 61 deaths in the Nottingham District in 1989. The two largest single killers in this group were accidents and respiratory disease. There were also significant differences between the sexes. All of the accidental deaths in those aged 5 to 14 were of boys.

In the age group from 15 to 44 years there were 201 deaths in Nottingham in 1989. Differences between the sexes are apparent in this age group too. As in the younger age group, the most common cause of death was accidents, of which nearly 80% were to men. The second leading cause of death was cancer, and about 66% of these fatal cancers were borne by women.

In the age group from 45 to 64 years there were 1093 deaths in 1989. In this age group cancer emerges as the leading cause of death. Forty-two per cent of all deaths in this age group were from cancer. It is this age group that heart disease too becomes a major killer, accounting for 32 per cent of all deaths. By contrast with the younger age groups, accidents account for only 4% of deaths in those aged 45–64 years.

In those over 64 years there were 5513 deaths in 1989. In this age band, heart disease takes over from cancer as the leading cause of death. This is followed by cancer, strokes and respiratory disease. In 1989, 80% of all deaths were in the 65 and over age group.

We have left until last deaths in those under 1 month of age. The cause of death in those under 1 month is difficult to establish and is not recorded. However, Nottingham's DPH notes in her report that perinatal mortality (deaths before and immediately after birth) had declined during the 1980s in Nottingham.

## THE USES OF MORTALITY DATA

On the one hand, mortality data are limited for the purposes of assessing the need for health care services. This is because mortality rates are affected not only by health care services but also by wider societal measures. On the other, mortality data are important because they allow us to monitor whether the population is becoming more healthy, but a healthier population is not the result solely of the provision of health care services. However, the DPH's breakdown of leading causes of death by age and sex is useful in enabling us to see clearly which age and sex groups are likely to benefit most from devoting resources to particular health problems. For example, resources devoted to the prevention of accidents may do much to reduce premature mortality in men but it will be of less benefit in reducing mortality in women and in the older age groups.

## MORBIDITY

It is far more difficult to obtain a picture of total morbidity (sickness and disease) than it is to obtain a picture of mortality. In part this is because it is less easy to define, quantify and measure such factors as pain, disability, and mental suffering than it is to measure death. There are difficulties too in obtaining relevant and appropriate information about morbidity. Much information about chronic ill-health, particularly conditions causing pain and disability but which do not require admission to hospital (e.g. arthritis) remains unrecorded. The DPH stresses that such information as exists on morbidity represents only the tip of a very large iceberg and much of the available information is not well-suited to the task of measuring the amount of morbidity that exists within the community. Often there is simply no information about a great deal of ill-health within the community. The DPH points to the danger in resource allocation of concentrating only on those conditions about which information exists. We would contend that those nurses, general practitioners and other health and community workers who often work in close proximity to individuals and families have a crucial role to play in drawing attention to much of this 'hidden' morbidity.

## OUTCOMES

Outcomes do not feature to a large extent in the Nottingham DHA reports from 1990 to 1995, at least in terms of setting goals for adding years to life, or life to years. In the 1993 report however the impact of the *Health of the Nation* White Paper published during the previous year can be seen. Referring to the targets set for the reduction of accidents in the Government's policy document the *Health of the Nation* (Department of Health 1992) the DPH refers to the *Health of the Nation* targets for a reduction in death rates as a result of accidents in each of three specific vulnerable groups: children under 15; young people aged 15–24; and people aged 65 and over. The DPH observes that proportionate reductions in deaths in Nottingham would result in modest reductions in mortality rates among the respective groups of people. However, she also makes the following statement on the prevention of accidents (Nottingham Health Authority 1993, p. 37): 'Whilst the targets (on accident prevention) are relatively simple to specify in principle, they are more difficult to achieve in practice, since they represent numerical indices which result from an interaction of many contributory factors. We need to move away from simplistic outcomes to address the more complex determinants involved'.

The DPH then refers to the work of a Nottingham Accident Prevention Group with 'representatives from a wide range of organizations' which had developed 'an excellent prevention strategy for the district' and whose key aims form the main recommendations for the section in the 1993 report on accidents. In this way the DPH neatly encapsulates the difficulties confronting a DHA in the reformed NHS after 1990. Apart from its specialized service for the surveillance, prevention, treatment and control of communicable diseases, the DHA is not a *provider* of services. It may therefore only improve the health of the district population for which it is responsible through its *influence* on other agencies, largely as a *purchaser* of their services. This indirect responsibility for health improvement is reflected throughout the Nottingham DPH reports in terms of recommendations which have more to do with the standard of services to be provided, or with the recurring reference to the need for an improvement in *information* in order to enhance the DHA's monitoring function.

## RESOURCES

Thus far we have tried to illustrate how one DPH tackled the complex task over a number of years of defining the health needs of one DHA. It has been seen that the assessment of health need relies on knowledge about mortality and morbidity rates, as well as knowledge about the factors which affect health which include age, sex, life-style, environment and the degree of deprivation. Health needs assessment also involves an assessment of the resources available to meet need. The example on accident prevention showed that resources include not only curative interventions and preventive and health promotion services, but also the organizational capability to bring together groups of people who can collectively begin to tackle the causes of the problem. An example of how this has worked in Nottingham lies in a road traffic policy where roads which were accident 'black spots' have been re-designed with 'sleeping policemen' in order to slow vehicles (see also Ch. 5). This could not have been achieved by the efforts of just one agency such as the DHA working alone, but instead has involved a whole range of community workers, including the police, transport department, as well as local health visitors and general practitioners. In this sense, Nottingham is demonstrating another of the *Health of the Nation* objectives in terms of setting up Healthy Alliances (Department of Health 1993b).

A strong focus of the Nottingham DPH reports is therefore on the *services* provided for the various populations whose needs are described. The most useful information about services concerns their effectiveness, that is, the ability of the population to benefit from services. Unfortunately, studies of effectiveness are relatively rare and this too is related to the complexity of the evaluation process.

The process which has been described illustrates how any health needs assessment exercise is shaped by the ultimate purpose for which it is intended, and this needs to be borne in mind when setting out to design an assessment. In Chapter 11, examples of how nursing students have carried out some form of health needs assessment as part of their course assessment will be presented. It is important to be clear therefore in terms of defining outcomes, whether this simply forms part of a learning process, or whether the finished products are designed ultimately to form part of a wider assessment strategy.

## CASE STUDY: CANCER

Before leaving the Nottingham DPH's reports, we discuss the assessment of the health needs of people with cancer (Nottingham Health Authority 1992). The approach adopted serves as a model for comprehensive local health needs assessment based on a disease category, at district level.

The DPH's assessment of the needs of people with cancer relies on knowledge about the following three things:

- the local level (incidence and prevalence) of cancer;
- the causes of cancer, including environmental and lifestyle factors;
- the resources to meet the needs of those with cancer.

All of these are included in the summary of the DPH's assessment which follows.

### The incidence and prevalence of cancer

Using the Trent Cancer Registry, the Nottingham Health Authority death register, and data from the Cancer Research Campaign the DPH is able to see which are the major types of cancer from which people suffer, and what the death and survival rates are for different cancers. Data from the OPCS also allow the DPH to examine the SMR for selected cancers in Nottingham.

The DPH is also able to look at the proportion of deaths from cancer as compared with deaths from other causes. In 1991, about a third of total deaths in Nottingham were from cancer. Cancer is a major cause of death in all adults, but especially in those aged 45–64, and especially in women. Although the *absolute* number of deaths from cancer is greater in the older age group, the *proportion* of deaths from cancer decreases in the older age group.

The DPH looks at premature mortality from cancer. On the assumption that people could be expected to live until the age of 75, she calculates the number of years of life lost as a result of cancer. Between 1985 and 1989 cancer resulted in 60 183 years of lost life as compared with 41 924 lost years of life from coronary heart disease. To reduce the number of these 'lost' years would meet the target of 'Adding Years to Life'.

Finally, the DPH stresses that demographic changes will affect the incidence and prevalence of cancer. About three-quarters of cancer deaths are in the over-65 age group, and as this age group grows larger so too will the number of cancer deaths.

## The causes of cancer

Not all of the causes of cancer are known. However, the causes of *some* cancers are well known. Cancer is very largely a preventable disease. The DPH quotes Sir Richard Doll (1992) who has suggested that, in the light of our present knowledge, the risk of developing cancer could in theory be reduced by 90%.

The DPH notes that some cancers have a genetic element. She also highlights three lifestyle factors associated with cancer: tobacco, diet and alcohol. Tobacco is responsible for about a third of all cancer deaths. The effect of diet is more difficult to ascertain but it has been estimated that diet plays a role in about 30% of cancers. The precise contribution of alcohol, too, is difficult to quantify but there is good evidence that alcohol compounds the effects of tobacco and diet.

## Resources to deal with cancer: primary prevention

The DPH stresses that prevention is not the responsibility only of the health care services. It is in part the responsibility of individuals themselves. However, individuals must be given real opportunities to adopt a healthier lifestyle. They must be provided with the right information. Moreover, the DPH suggests that shopkeepers should be encouraged by public and professional demand to stock a much wider range of cheap, high-fibre, low-fat foods.

## Screening

Any health care intervention, preventive or curative, must have demonstrable benefits which outweigh its costs, and must be acceptable to the people it is intended to benefit (see Ch. 8). Screening is one type of intervention in which clear criteria have been developed against which particular screening programmes can be evaluated. The DPH states that before a screening programme for cancer is introduced both the disease and the programme should be evaluated against the following criteria, which have been examined in greater depth in Chapter 8 (Burr & Elwood 1991):

- the disease should be common and serious;

- there should be a long period before symptoms develop when the disease may be identified and treated;
- early treatment of the disease must be better than later treatment;
- the test should be simple to apply to large numbers of people;
- the test should be acceptable to most people, for example, not inconvenient or uncomfortable and without ill-effects;
- the test should be able reliably to identify people with the disease and exclude those who do not have the disease.

## Genetic screening

Population screening for genetic abnormalities which predispose to cancer is not yet possible, but technological developments may soon make this possible. The DPH notes that such developments will bring in their train many ethical issues, for example in relation to individuals' ability to obtain insurance and employment. She argues that local and national community involvement at an early stage is essential if technology is not to outpace ethical considerations.

## Breast screening

Nottingham, in line with the National Breast Screening Programme, is currently undertaking breast screening in women aged 50–64 where there is evidence, based on national studies, that screening can lead to the prolongation of life and a reduction in mortality. The National Screening Programme expects to prevent about 25% of deaths from breast cancer in those who are screened. The DPH notes that it is too early to see what the effect of the programme will be in Nottingham.

## Cervical screening

There is evidence that cervical screening programmes are also effective. However, there is also evidence that those women most at risk of cervical cancer are least likely to attend for screening. Nottingham has a cervical screening programme and rates of attendance for screening are high, although rates of cervical cancer are also high.

## Cancer of the large bowel

It is not known whether a screening programme for cancer of the large bowel would be effective. A large trial is currently being carried out in Nottingham to investigate its effectiveness.

Finally, the DPH notes that screening programmes have personal and resource implications. Screening can lead to anxiety and there must be follow-up services both to counsel those undergoing screening tests and to ensure that the abnormalities detected can be dealt with.

## Cancer diagnosis and treatment

The majority of treatments for cancer have never been formally evaluated, and there are few data available concerning their impact of patients. This, the DPH stresses, requires urgent remedy.

## Hospital care

The DPH notes that the majority of people with cancer in Nottingham spend most of their illness at home or elsewhere in the community, although over 60% die in hospital. Much hospital care is not curative. A study of people with terminal cancer showed that people were admitted to hospital for three main reasons: 40% for control of symptoms, 27% for support as they lacked family or other carers to support them at home, and finally because they lacked social services support. The DPH notes that such patients do not always have their needs fully met in hospital. She highlights, too, an urgent need for closer liaison between all the people, services and specialties involved in cancer care.

## Palliative care

Palliative care involves several elements:

- relief from pain and other distressing symptoms;
- psychological and spiritual care;
- a support system for patients;
- a support system for patients' families and other carers.

The DPH notes that in relation to palliative care the definition of need employed by the DHA and by service providers may differ from the views of patients and carers (Nottingham Health Authority 1992). It is vital in this area to consider the views of patients and their families when defining their needs.

Palliative care is provided in a range of settings including specialist in-patient units, hospices, nursing homes and patients' own homes. The DPH notes that palliative care services in Nottingham are not meeting the amount of need for such care that exists in the community.

The DPH recognizes that not all patients will eventually die at home or in a hospice and she therefore urges that the highest standard of terminal care must be made available in all settings, and all health workers in contact with those who are dying must be appropriately trained. The DPH urges that the quality of care, with specific standards of care for the dying, must be promoted through the contracting process with service providers.

## Home care

The majority of deaths from cancer occur in people over 65, and many of these people live alone or have spouses who, too, are old and may be ill. The DPH believes a fundamental policy of cancer care must be that patients should always be able to remain at home if they so chose. This means that an intensive nursing service must be available in the home setting. The DPH notes that such a service is not always available to Nottingham residents and she believes that the development of such a service should be a high priority.

## Respite care

The DPH notes that currently in Nottingham there are only a small number of services providing respite care, and that the needs of patients and carers for respite care are not being fully met.

## Collaboration between providers; coordination of care, and inter-agency co-operation

Palliative care is provided by a range of specialists in the public and private sectors. There is a need for greater collaboration between provider units. There is a need also for better collaboration and planning between purchasers – the DHA and the local authority. Finally, there is a need to plan the care of each patient instead of responding to problems on an ad hoc basis. GPs and community nurses are well placed to plan and co-ordinate care but are often not given the information they need by hospital staff. Improved communication links are therefore identified as necessary for improved service effectiveness.

## The needs of carers

Caring can be a lonely and frightening experience. The DPH believes that the needs of carers should always be separately assessed.

Support and counselling from caring agencies can be of tremendous benefit.

## Cultural and religious needs

On the basis of a review carried out by the public health department, the DPH was made aware that the differing cultures of patients and their carers are not always being respected. She was disturbed to discover that some services were not being taken up for this reason. She stresses that it is vital to be aware of the cultural and religious needs of patients. Staff must be trained in race awareness and information must be available in appropriate languages and styles. Dietary needs must be responded to, too.

## Complementary therapies

Finally, the DPH stresses that people should be able to choose whatever treatments they feel may help them in addition to mainstream treatments. Few GPs and other professionals are aware of the existing range of complementary therapies, and evidence of their efficacy is lacking. The DPH suggest that the DHA and the Family Health Services Authority should attempt to remedy this.

## Recommendations

The DPH makes several recommendations. As in the case of accidents discussed above, these recommendations relate predominantly to standards of care which the DHA will be concerned to incorporate and monitor in any purchasing agreement (Nottingham Health Authority 1992):

- hospice standards of care should be promoted for all patients during their final illness irrespective of where they are cared for;
- patients must be supported to remain at home throughout their illness if they wish. Home care should be a priority in developing new services;
- an intensive home nursing service, easily accessible to all who need it, should be afforded a high priority;
- providers and personnel in different provider units should collaborate more closely;
- purchasers should collaborate to develop shared plans for palliative services;

- new treatments must be fully evaluated before they are introduced.

## CONCLUSION

It can be seen from the above case study just how comprehensive a full health needs assessment needs to be from a purchasing authority's point of view. Not everyone carrying out health needs assessment will be so inclusive. For example, health visitors developing a case load profile will include data predominantly from their own case load in order to define their potential workload and to monitor their success in covering the health needs within it. This will be a more limited exercise, although still essential if the service provided is to be effectively planned, prioritized and monitored.

# Health profiling by nurses

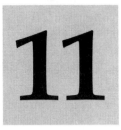

## CONTENTS

## INTRODUCTION

Numerous excellent studies on local health needs assessment carried out by practising community nurses as well as by student health visitors, district nurses, school nurses, midwives and pre-registration nurses, have been carried out locally in the past. Regrettably, because nurses traditionally have not enjoyed a good record of publishing their work, much of this work has never been privileged to see the light of day in terms of a wider audience. This chapter is an attempt to portray the essence of some small part of this activity. It begins with reference to research commissioned by the English National Board (ENB) into consumer views on the nature of needs assessment in primary health care which forms part of a larger study into the educational needs of community nurses. The findings from this research reinforce the account of health needs assessment as part of a *process* similar to that reported in the second part of the chapter which describes the Public Health health visiting function developed in the Strelley Nursing Development (health visiting) Unit (NDU) at Nottingham. Finally, the chapter concludes with extracts from some of the Neighbourhood Studies carried out by first and second year undergraduate nurses on the Bachelor of Nursing (Hons) course at

Nottingham. These studies demonstrate the types of preparation for health needs assessment which is being carried out as part of degree level Project 2000 pre-registration nurse education courses. The evidence presented in this chapter is by its nature mainly local and selective. It raises however the larger question 'How much similar work is going on around the country that is neither disseminated nor used?'

## HEALTH NEEDS ASSESSMENT BY COMMUNITY NURSES

Practising nurses, midwives and health visitors have several advantages when carrying out locally-based health needs assessment.

First, they are not restricted to looking only at health problems. Like Frankenberg's anthropologists working in Africa (see Ch. 1) community nurses are *participants* and the advantage of the health needs assessment exercises which they carry out is that they incorporate not only health and social *problems* but also aspects of a local community's *strengths*. For example, an area of social deprivation may also be characterized by a strong sense of local identity and it may therefore be easier to form local community groups. This aspect of community life was identified in the Strelley NDU and several of the neighbourhood studies carried out by undergraduate nurses in areas of social deprivation. Local groups may take the form of semi-permanent organizations such as tenants' associations, or more loosely structured networks such as women's groups, either of which may take on issues in order to work collectively for some common objective. If community nurses have a sense of both an area's strengths *and* problems they are far more likely to be able to contribute to realistic local policies (see reference to Community Profiling at Strelley below). This is a much more comprehensive, 'bottom up' approach than when DHAs and Local Authorities look *separately* at health and social problems, for no such separation of experience exists for the families and communities where practising nurses work on a daily basis.

Second, nurses working in the community have the further advantage that they are in direct day to day touch with many patients, clients and community representatives, and with the individual professional colleagues who go to make up the inter-sectoral (or inter-agency) groups which the Department of Health urges to work together as part of the *Health of the Nation* strategy. Their assessments will therefore contribute much which is of direct relevance to local people.

Third, practising nurses have first hand experience of how government policies actually impact on the client groups for whom they were intended. Sometimes policies implemented with the best of intentions can have unintended consequences. An example is shown in the findings of the small but important empirical study referred to in the introduction, on how consumers viewed the government's proposals for health needs assessment following the 1990 NHS Health and Community Care Act. Cowley et al (1994) report that consumers were very critical of the notion of 'need' as something which suggested that one was 'needy' or 'demanding'. This is an interesting perspective from the consumer's point of view, given that health economists frequently use the terms 'need' and 'demand' in the specialist language of their academic discipline. One respondent explained the subtle difference: 'Maybe if I went to somebody and said "I need . . . " that might get their back up, but if I was to go there and say "I'd like . . . " or "could you help me . . . " in a certain way, not "I need"'. Those interviewed by Cowley et al were highly sceptical of the motives behind 'top down' notions of needs assessment. The following extract from the interviews suggests that policy guidance on how to assess needs is unduly prescriptive and bureaucratic; in contrast to community nurses' much more informal, traditional ways of working (Cowley et al 1994):

> Our health visitor came in and she's got a form about as thick as that and she starts 'I just want to ask you a few questions if you don't mind dear, now is this your second baby and now, have you ever been sexually abused?' Well no; and then we've got, 'Do you have a drug problem?' Meaning, you know, do you take cocaine, crack, do you inject heroin intravenously? Well no; 'Do you have an alcohol problem? Was your childhood happy or did your father beat you senseless and lock you in a cupboard for three days?' You know, if I'd been sneaking off into the kitchen to take crack cocaine, I don't think I would have told her when she asked me for this form, but then they go away from the area saying right these parents are all very nice . . . . . . . they don't have any needs. So you never see them again.

It appears, at least from this respondent, that people resent being categorised on a 'once and for all basis' and that they prefer community workers who are not tied to the dictates of an investigative bureaucracy. This perspective is supported by the contention of Hawtin et al that community profiling should be comprehensive and challenge 'bureaucratic departmentalism' (see Ch. 9).

Respondents in the study of Cowley et al were also 'wary of the idea that needs assessment should be something separate from service provision and that it should take account of the needs of both the "cared for" and the "carer"'. Concern was expressed that needs assessment should not simply become a 'number crunching' exercise subject to the need to 'fit the budget, rather than the other way round'. Cowley et al suggest that by contrast with the contemporary separation of the assessment from sebsequent service delivery, community nurses have tried traditionally to take a personal-subjective dimension into account; treating assessment as an individualized *process* which was *not* a 'once and for all' statement but part of an ongoing relationship between the nurse and the client.

The situation is not all gloomy. Cowley et al (1994) reported that their research in progress suggested that where community nurses were moving towards a case management approach to practice, assessment was proving to be a key function of the role, and they give examples of good practice (Boyd 1993, Gilbert 1993). This perspective also comes through from the accounts of the health needs assessment process carried out as part of the Strelley NDU's Public Health health visiting activities at Nottingham described below.

## HEALTH NEEDS ASSESSMENT BY HEALTH VISITORS: STRELLEY NDU

The Strelley Nursing Development Unit's (Health Visiting) first Annual Report 1992–93 sets out the philosophy and aims for the provision of health visiting in an area of social deprivation, which includes health needs assessment as one of its methods. The report states (Nottingham Community Health NHS Trust 1993, p. 1):

> The philosophy of Strelley NDU is 'The people in Strelley have the right to high quality preventative health care, that is relevant, acceptable, equitable and accessible.' The focus . . . . has been around Health Visiting assessment and increasing the service's accessibility to the local population. Much of the development work has been related to profiling and prioritizing health visiting work by identifying health needs and

exposing unmet needs. Subsequently we hope to clarify the role of Health Visitors working in an area of social deprivation and poor health status. This information will be the basis for targeting future work in line with *Health of the Nation* and Nottingham's health strategy.

One of the developments to come out of the Strelley NDU was the establishment of Public Health health visiting practice from which a number of projects were developed, for example (Boyd et al 1993, p. 10):

- Strelley accident prevention group, an example of a 'healthy alliance' of a variety of workers and local people relating to a national (*Health of the Nation*) target;
- the women's health and leisure group, formed in response to locally identified need and run by local people for themselves;
- a 'No Smoking Day', an initiative prompted by a national campaign, and involving a wide range of local health staff.

Part of the Public Health health visitor role was to collect and co-ordinate information on the local population's health status in the form of a Community Profile. The profile drew on a range of information from sources which included: the DHA Public Health Department, Health Visiting profiles (all health visitors in Nottingham carry out case load profiles which include information on family employment and income support based on the recommendations of Blackburn 1992a), County Council Planning and Transportation, and Road Safety Departments, Nottingham City Council Housing Department, Family Health Services Authority and the NSPCC. The profile focussed on the level of poverty and its impact on family health and well being. It included Standardized Mortality Rates and Unemployment figures by ward, and locally collected data such as waiting lists for nursery provision and other local resources.

The Strelley NDU's Annual Report 1994 (the penultimate year that the Unit received support funding from the King's Fund Nursing Development Unit budget) set out some of the Unit's achievements (Nottingham Community Health NHS Trust 1994). Poverty is seen as central to the Strelley team's public health concerns and poverty indicators are documented and updated regularly. For example, the report cited an unemployment rate of 23.5% in Strelley in September 1993, compared with 11.9% in the UK as a whole. The evidence which had been collected suggests that 'Deprivation is associated with many health and social problems and the team's health profiling, based on poverty indicators, enabled it to target resources at the most "needy" within a deprived area' (Nottingham Community Health NHS Trust, 1994, p. 5). In looking to the way forward, the Strelley team identifies the need to continue work on health visiting outcomes, specifically exploring the benefits for the local population. The team had already identified indicators arising from targets set in *A Vision for the Future* (NHS Management Executive 1993a), including immunization rates and uptake of development assessment for children, and they had established baseline data for other targets, such as a reduction in teenage pregnancies.

The Strelley NDU implicitly incorporated three elements of health needs assessment referred to in Chapter 9 – health (and social) problems, resources, and outcomes. Although acutely aware of the higher SMRs in the area in which they worked, the Strelley health visitors' idea of outcomes was much more oriented to health gain in the form of adding 'life to years' than merely adding 'years to life'. They frequently found themselves working towards these goals 'against the grain'. In describing *Public Health at Strelley: a Model in Action*, Brummell & Perkins (1995, p. 2) state:

> The NDU and the public health post were set up in a political environment which is comparatively unfavourable to this kind of work. The individualistic ideology supported by the Conservative Government has resulted in the progressive rolling back of the welfare state; there is now more emphasis on individuals' responsibility to care for their own health, and less on the role of structural constraints in limiting the health choices available to individuals, or the responsibility of the state to increase these choices.

Yet in this relatively unfavourable environment much was achieved. Twenty-two projects based on responses to locally expressed need were eventually carried out with people in the local community. Above all, at a time of budgetary constraint in the service and relatively high levels of poverty amongst the local population, Strelley NDU managed to increase both material and information resources for health. Multi-agency working increased and completely innovative health-promoting schemes flourished. In addition to all of this activity the group also managed to publish their work. It is by their struggle to fulfil their commitment to dissemination (unlike so much good work carried out by community nurses in the past) that the Strelley

NDU experiment will continue to be referred to and replicated by community nursing staff.

## HEALTH NEEDS ASSESSMENT: THE LEARNING EXPERIENCE

In the Foreword to this book the shift to a community health-based model of nurse education following the introduction of the Project 2000 reforms is described. One consequence of this shift is that student nurses begin to learn about health before disease, and usually experience their first practice placements in the community. Like the description of the achievements of the Strelley NDU above, this section of the chapter is also drawn from locally based experience, in this case derived from the teaching of health needs assessment to undergraduates on a four year Bachelor of Nursing (BN) course. Because of the health and community orientation of Project 2000 courses, health needs assessment comes early in the teaching on the Nottingham BN and forms the basis for an assignment known as the Neighbourhood Study. The philosophy behind the Nottingham BN Neighbourhood Study embodies the following principles:

1. The Neighbourhood Study provides an ideal vehicle for self-directed learning concerning issues of health and healing in the community.

2. Carrying out the Neighbourhood Study is a gradual process of learning and reflecting on:
    (a) the many factors which influence the health of individuals and groups, and
    (b) the part that various services (health, local authority, voluntary and private sector) may, or may not, contribute to that health status.

3. The lessons learned from carrying out the Study enable a transfer of learning to take place so that they may be applied at any time, in any place.

4. There is no such thing as a standard Neighbourhood Study. Every one will be different – even those carried out in the same geographical area. This is the student's study!

5. There is considerable freedom of choice as to the subject selected

for study and its ultimate presentation (subject to the usual rider about consultation with tutor).

This project-based piece of work is in two parts consisting first of a 1000-word structured Neighbourhood Study Plan which sets out the aim(s), objectives and proposed action for completion of the Neighbourhood Study itself. The Plan is submitted during the second semester in Year 1 of the course. The Plan has the following objectives:

1. To set out a logical structure for the work leading up the eventual submission of the Neighbourhood Study, including a time frame.

2. To select a particular geographical 'Neighbourhood' for the study of a particular area of health need and/or service provision, and to justify that selection.

3. To discuss, with reference to appropriate literature, the expected strengths and weaknesses of selecting a small geographical area (neighbourhood) for health needs assessment.

4. To select a particular focus for the study of health needs assessment and/or service provision and describe the reasons for that selection.

5. To describe the various sources of information to which access will be sought in order to complete the Neighbourhood Study, with a brief description of their expected strengths and limitations.

Preparation for the Plan requires that the students begin to think critically about the definitions of terms such as 'neighbourhood' and 'community' which are frequently used in everyday language to imply different or imprecise meanings. The fourth objective, to select a particular focus, is designed to ensure that the student does not just *describe* a particular geographical area, but also considers the needs of, and resources available to, a particular group of people, or services, in the community. Students are also required to identify the sources of information which will be needed in order to complete the Study. They are reminded that information may be derived from:

- formal sources such as government, local authority and DHA publications;
- library sources for information on policy issues and on the topic chosen for their particular focus;
- local sources such as GP lists and practice profiles, reports written

by professional or community groups, parish magazines, brochures and sources of local history often found in the local library;

- informal sources such as observations gathered from professionals, and clients and patients during practice placements.

Issues concerning the reliability, generalizability and confidentiality of the different sources of information are discussed. Students are not permitted to carry out surveys in order to complete the Study for three reasons. First, the exercise is intended to demonstrate the availability, volume and range of pre-existing material for use in health needs assessment. Second, students have not received research methods training at this stage in their course. Third, the exercise should be relatively unobtrusive and should not overload the community with numerous requests for access to new sources of information.

Students are encouraged before they go out on their first community placement to reflect on the following issues:

- what do the terms 'neighbourhood' and 'community' mean from their own personal experiences and from sources in the literature?
- is a neighbourhood the same as a community?
- what factors need to be taken into account in order to be able to describe somewhere as a neighbourhood?
- what might the student be looking for when describing
  (a) the health needs of a neighbourhood?
  (b) neighbourhood health services?

The 2500–3000 word Neighbourhood Study itself is submitted at the end of semester 3 in Year 2 of the course and comprises an essay building on the Plan and describing:

- The student's assessment of a particular neighbourhood identified during their community placements;
- An assessment of a particular area of health need and/or service provision investigated within the context of that particular neighbourhood.

The following section gives some examples of the work carried out for the Neighbourhood Studies.

## NEIGHBOURHOOD STUDIES: SOME EXAMPLES OF STUDENTS' LOCAL HEALTH NEEDS ASSESSMENTS

The following extracts are selected from a sample of twelve studies completed between 1992 and 1994. The studies were selected for the way in which students had chosen to address issues in health needs assessment, including the lessons which they claimed to have learnt from carrying out the study. The chosen studies tended to have amongst the highest marks in the range for their years but this was not the prime reason for the selection which was to demonstrate the variety of issues and methods of presentation. The selection of findings from the studies will be presented under the headings identified in Chapter 9 on health needs assessment at the local level:

population and health needs definition and selection;
comprehensiveness;
resources;
outcomes.

## POPULATION AND HEALTH NEEDS: DEFINITION AND SELECTION

Nottingham DHA consists of five local government administrative districts: Nottingham City, Broxtowe, Gedling, Hucknall, and Rushcliffe. Student community placements tend to be shared around these districts and this is reflected in the following proportions of geographical neighbourhoods included in the twelve studies listed in Table 11.1.

Although students identified electoral wards for the purposes of examining census data for their chosen populations, they noted that administrative geographical boundaries are only of limited use when considering the needs of local populations. Six of the twelve studies (including three in the City) referred to neighbourhoods based on traditional village or small town names which bore no relationship to the electoral ward(s) in which they were based. None of the students selected the same health need for the focus of their study and their choice was wide-ranging:

**Table 11.1** Twelve studies in the Nottingham District Health Authority area

| District | Number of studies | Number of wards |
|---|---|---|
| Nottingham City | 7 | 10 |
| Broxtowe | 2 | 7 |
| Gedling | – | – |
| Hucknall | – | – |
| Rushcliffe | 3 | 5 |
| Total | 12 | 22 |

1. The health needs of lone mothers
2. Maternity facilities for young, single, pregnant women living in hostels
3. Child care facilities for single mothers
4. Children with learning disabilities
5. Accommodation for the elderly
6. Health and the health needs of the elderly
7. Diabetes in the elderly
8. The needs of carers
9. Homelessness and health needs
10. Unemployment and health
11. Health promotion and education with reference to HIV and AIDS
12. Screening services for breast and cervical cancer

Students will be identified by the above numbers when reporting findings from the studies. The following extracts are selected as small case studies to demonstrate some of the issues which the students identified. Some rich material is inevitably omitted. Because students tended to collapse discussion of the identification of a 'neighbourhood' together with their chosen topic, the two categories of population and health needs definition and selection are also collapsed in the following account.

## Homelessness

Students observed that geographical boundaries are of very limited use when considering certain health needs scenarios. For example, in relation to homelessness, Student 9 wrote:

To an extent, the difficulty of defining a neighbourhood is less of an issue when considering people who are homeless because they are transient, and do not all live in one definable area. There is a pattern in the degree of homelessness found in my chosen area, however. The size of the homeless population varies as one travels along the main road. It is most severe closest to (the city), decreasing as one moves closer to (a village) and the countryside. There is little evidence of the homeless outside the city centre during the day-time, suggesting that it is very much a hidden phenomenon.

Student 9 identified different classifications of homelessness and reported the legal definition of 'homelessness' in the Housing (Homeless Persons) Act 1985, Part III. She noted that being single and homeless is a particular difficulty because familied homeless are given higher priority in terms of temporary accommodation. Student 9 established that there were between 250 and 300 street and shelter homeless in Nottingham and that their most immediate needs were for health services, housing, money and food, and she identified that Nottingham has a dedicated health care team for the homeless which attempts to meet their needs in acceptable and appropriate ways.

## Screening

In relation to GP based screening (see Ch. 8), Student 12 noted the overlap of GP populations in an inner city area which makes the identification of a denominator extremely difficult: 'Six practices are classified as being part of the "X" ward, with a total population for cervical screening of 1158'. Nevertheless, ward-based data were still useful in helping Student 12 to identify the characteristics of material deprivation experienced in the neighbourhood: '"X" ward has a score on the Jarman index of 56.7 (range −46, affluent, to +58 deprived) and 10 on the Townsend index (range −6, affluent, to +11 deprived).....Material and social deprivation also stems from having the highest unemployment rate, exceeding 40% (Department of Employment, and Nottinghamshire County Council 1993)'. Student 12 was interested in trying to identify whether, in the face of such deprivation, uptake of screening services for local women was lower than average (as she understood had been reported by the *Black Report* (Townsend & Davidson 1992; see also Ch. 5). In relation to the ward's female population she reported that:

.... they not only experience the deprivation resulting from unemployment and low incomes, but as women they are subjected to a number of unique social forces. *Poverty in Nottingham* (Nottingham City

Council 1994) claims that within Nottingham, 94% of lone parent households are headed by women. Four times as many women as men work part-time, 79% of those being low paid. It is often seen as women's natural role to take responsibility for childcare and domestic duties. This places many women in extremely stressful situations. With little money, they must feed, clothe and care for their children, and at the same time live their own lives.

Having examined the rationale behind breast and cervical screening, and its provision in the practice in which she did her community placement, Student 12 identified that uptake for local women, while below national and regional targets, was higher than anticipated, being respectively 43% and 65%. She concluded her study with an examination of the literature on non-uptake and made recommendations for improvement in the area of her neighbourhood study. Many of the recommendations were administrative, including the need for the practice to improve its methods of communication and record keeping so that local women who tended to be geographically mobile within the area were not lost to screening because appointments went to the wrong address. She also saw a need for the members of the primary health care team to improve their educational roles in order to convey essential information, allay anxiety, and to ensure that test results were followed up and understood.

## Accommodation for the elderly

The benefits of closely examining ward-based census data emerged when Student 5 was still deciding on her choice of topic; she wrote:

By consulting the data from the 1991 census it is possible to construct a picture of the local population within the neighbourhood (2 wards comprising a village). The total population is 6482, 48% male and 52% female. When we look more closely at the neighbourhood's population, we can detect discrepancies. For example, the (proportion of the rural) district's under 16 population is 18.9%, for my neighbourhood this figure is only 16.95%. The neighbourhood is also under-represented in the 16–24 and 25 to pensionable age groups. When looking at the elderly population we can understand why. The 2 wards have a total of 1410 people who are of pensionable age, this represents about 21.7% of their (total) population. In relation to the district's 18.5% we can see why (the neighbourhood). would have needs (relating to the elderly) inconsistent with surrounding neighbourhoods . . . . . This over-respresentation of the elderly was one of my reasons for studying this group further, to see whether (the village) was meeting the needs of its elderly population, or if there were major gaps in service provision.

Student 5 also observed on her placement with a district nurse mentor that many of the people visited on her caseload were in residential care. She wrote:

> .... in (the village) alone there were eight different (types of accommodation) available for the over 65s, including psycho-geriatric, nursing homes, private residential care and warden-aided housing. Even though the emphasis is now upon keeping the elderly in their own homes and supporting them through community care, I felt that as (the village's) residential figures were extraordinarily high, it would be interesting to look into the choice available for those needing to enter it.

During the process of her study, Student 5 identified many subtle aspects to the provision of residential care for the elderly and that, despite the apparently abundant provision, there were still gaps in local services. Many of the elderly people visited during her visits with the district nurse were unaware that homes could sometimes be used for respite care, and most people still living in their own homes held extremely negative views of residential care. Student 5 felt therefore that considerable improvements in information provision could be made if there was a more coordinated approach by local community workers.

## The needs of carers

In looking at the needs of carers in a 'neighbourhood' consisting of a small town comprising three wards, Student 8 was confronted with problems of defining a 'carer' and also how to count them. On definition, Student 8 wrote: 'A carer is someone whose life is in some way restricted by the need to be responsible for the care of someone who is mentally ill, mentally handicapped or whose health is impaired by sickness or old age (Pitkeathley 1989)'. Student 8 also identified that the term 'informal carer' is sometimes used to distinguish carers from professional health workers. She felt that this belittles the role of carers and spoke to several who felt the term implicitly ignored the major scarifices and commitment they make in order to fulfil their role.

In order to gain some idea of how many carers there might be in her neighbourhood, Student 8 extrapolated from national statistics in order to gain a picture of how many carers there were likely to be in the town. Data from the 1990 General Household Survey suggested that there were about 6.8 million carers in Great Britain, a quarter of whom spend 20 hours or more a week on caring activities. Four per cent of adults cared for someone living in the same household.

Extrapolations from these figures suggest there were likely to be over 2500 people in Student 8's neighbourhood providing some degree of care, and over 800 people looking after a dependant in the same household. The study was also able to ascertain that the number of carers in Nottingham looked set to increase. National data showed that the majority of people being cared for are over 65 and that the elderly population is increasing.

Student 8 discussed the main problems facing carers under the headings: loneliness and isolation; carers' own health (which was generally poor but they believed that GPs were reluctant to find anything wrong with them as they were needed to care for the dependent person); information; and support. She found that the carers she spoke to did not mention the problems of guilt and stigma which had been identified in the literature as associated with caring for someone who manifests anti-social behaviour. This may have been because of embarrassment, and Student 8 recommended that this should be taken into consideration when considering provision for carers as the literature describes a vicious circle of social withdrawal, loss of friends and social support.

Student 8 was highly critical of the provision of support for carers in the neighbourhood which she studied. She found that the objective of the 1990 NHS and Community Care Act to make practical support for carers a high priority was not being met by either health or social services. Student 8 found that the two most useful services identified by carers (a Care Attendant Scheme and a Caring and Sharing Group) were funded by voluntary contributions, charitable donations and a special Joint Finance Grant. Student 8 concluded:

> ... it is not enough to accept the problem or just quantify it. Action is required. There is a role for all statutory services in this action. Quality information must be readily available; the illnesses of dependent people must be de-stigmatized to enable more carers to come forward for help; health care professionals must recognize the needs of the carer and be prepared to share the burden; and opportunities for respite care that suit the needs of the carer must be made available.

## COMPREHENSIVENESS

Even though the students are required to focus on a particular topic for their study, the majority were comprehensive in their approach to issues. Comprehensiveness could be described in two ways. First, a *horizontal* approach where a particular topic was described in broad terms. Several students pointed out that health needs assessment applies to all aspects of health which includes physical, mental, social and emotional aspects.

## Health needs of the elderly

Student 6, drawing on Smyth (1992), saw that the needs of the elderly were not defined narrowly but included physical needs, functional needs, emotional needs, social needs, occupational needs, spiritual needs and health needs. Meeting needs was thus seen to be dependent on a range of physical, emotional and social factors including a healthy diet, good housing which is safe and comfortable, an acceptable standard of living, good health, emotional security, and leisure interests and socializing (Windmall 1992). Student 6 concluded:

> Perhaps the most important and effective service has been left to last – informal care which is provided by community carers and family and friends. The extent of this support system for the elderly varies widely. Most support comes from the spouse of immediate family . . . . . . However with an increasing proportion of the very old, there are fewer spouses left alive, and the children who might provide care may themselves be in their late fifties or sixties. . . . . . . I feel that without this support, individuals could be impoverished and immobilized.

## Children with learning disabilities

Similarly, Student 4 in looking at the needs of children with learning disabilities, suggested that most publications refer to the needs of both the child *and* the family, and that these include, in addition to the need for access to health services and respite care, the need for counselling, advice, and social help and support. (See also Student 4's observations in relation to outcomes below.)

## Unemployment and health

Student 10 examined unemployment and health in relation to a village where the local pit had recently closed. According to her interpretation of comprehensiveness, she drew a very definite connection between economic issues and the identification of health needs, saying:

> Overall there needs to be a greater awareness of the health dimension to economic and social change. Arguably, whilst the government gives health on one hand it takes it away with the other. The *Health of the Nation* strategy without doubt is a positive awareness of health, however, the abrupt pit closure programme and the deprivation it causes has

enormous negative health implications. As the RCN highlights, individuals only have so much 'choice' over health issues, and policies must 'create the right climate for people to make healthy choices' (Royal College of Nursing 1991b, p. 4). Unemployment, as a social situation, is a fundamental example of this.

Student 10 also identified that it is important to be wary of attributing a mythical 'community spirit' to areas of social deprivation with the sometimes mistaken idea that this helps local people band together for mutual support. Referring to a conversation with the local vicar with whom she had talked about the pit closure, Student 10 observed: 'Newspaper articles from the time of the pit closure presented the village as a united front fighting the proposals. According to local people, it was a time of hope that pulled the community together. Now it appears that the community has become fragmented into "who has and hasn't got a job".'

A second use of the term 'comprehensiveness' relates to the *vertical* approach to data and information. Many of the students included in their studies data not only from official sources such as Census information, General Household Survey and local reports on poverty, but also information collected locally from clients and patients, community nurses and GPs. They needed to be careful not to generalize from local information and to be extremely discrete in ensuring the confidentiality of their sources. That said, the local information greatly enriched the students' accounts and helped to convey the feeling that they had grasped a real sense of aspects of the local community and what it meant 'to listen to local voices' (NHS Management Executive 1992).

## Health promotion and education in HIV and AIDS

Student 11's study of health promotion and education in relation to HIV and AIDS proved to be very difficult to carry out in terms of obtaining local information on the prevalence and incidence of these conditions. In part this was because of the confidentiality of information where the numbers of people actually diagnosed as having AIDS within the DHA as a whole was very small, and non-existent in the neighbourhood studied. (1991 was the last year that data were available when this student was carrying out her study in 1993–94.) In part, it was also recognized that existing statistics are likely to be an underestimate because of under-reporting, use of services outside the district, and a number of individuals who may be HIV-positive but remain asymptomatic.

At one level, therefore, Student 11 felt that she had been remarkably *unsuccessful* in achieving her objectives, but this was because of the nature of the subject on which she had chosen to focus. Student 11's achievement lay in the picture which she was able to convey of local professional worker's *attitudes* to AIDS. She identified that Health and Sex Education had been delegated as a part of the National Curriculum to her mentor, the School Nurse for the local comprehensive school. However, the nurse had no control over the stage in the school curriculum at which she was allowed to teach, and in her view the sessions came too late in the young people's school life. Teachers were reluctant to become involved, even though the vast majority of parents were prepared for their children to attend these sessions. There were also limits imposed by the Headteacher as to what the School Nurse was allowed to include in relation to 'safer sex'.

Conversation with the local GP also revealed the difficulties in which local doctors may find themselves. He felt that when young girls come for their first contraceptive advice they may be too embarrassed to talk openly about the topic of HIV and AIDS, especially as this is not what they came to see the doctor about. It was his view that there should be a much more well directed media approach to this age group, supported by government. Thus, Student 11 identified at a local level just how ambivalent are our attitudes to preventive strategies in HIV and AIDS. Only the School Nurse appeared to be prepared to engage in health education appropriate to the young people's needs for information and at appropriate stages of their development. However, she was constrained by policies in other sectors and appeared powerless to influence policy in such a sensitive area.

## RESOURCES

All students discussed resources in the sense of the availability of local services and whether or not they met the needs of the group on whom they had chosen to focus. Resources were seen both in the widest sense of community resources overall, and in the specific sense of resources for particular needs. Community resources were seen to be especially important for groups who experienced material and social deprivation.

### Health and social resources for lone mothers

Students 1–3 studied some aspect of single motherhood in three different areas of social deprivation and remarkable similarities were found between their resource needs. Student 3 found a direct relationship between single mothers' poverty, their lack of access to education and training, and the non-availability of affordable child care facilities, and she observed:

> After speaking to people in the Health Centre it became evident that there is a general lack of support networks for single parents. A particularly distressing case was that of a young, single, mother who had been rejected by her family and could not see any way to improve her situation without gaining access to free child care facilities. This illustrates the need for more support, such as nursery places for the children of mothers wishing to work.

Student 2 who studied the maternity needs of single, pregnant mothers living in hostels found that a considerable level of health and voluntary service provision exists for single mothers in Nottingham in terms of 'drop-in' centres, and support and information concerning pregnancy, parenting and individual problems. In common with Student 3, the intractable problems for mothers in temporary accommodation centred around their difficulties in being able to obtain and maintain any form of employment. Several women had given up jobs in bars and fast food restaurants because a nightly 'curfew' operated in the hostel. Thus, one mother who had her flat re-possessed because of rent arrears, found it very difficult to pay off her debts.

Student 1 also found that lone mothers' greatest problems arose from their lack of education, skills and training and a reported general sense of low esteem. The mothers in her study tended, on the whole, to have better extended family support than those in the studies of Students 2 and 3. Also, the neighbourhood had several community centres running fitness classes, self-defence, swimming clubs, play groups and mother and toddler groups. Nevertheless, despite these levels of community and family support, it was observed (in common with Student 10's study of unemployment in a mining village) that health in its widest sense is related to a large extent to an individual's ability to engage in economic activity. Thus, all of the students who studied aspects of an area's social deprivation observed at first hand just how important is the relationship between material resources and the ability to participate fully in society as a social being.

## Diabetes in the elderly

Students also observed specific resource needs in relation to health and social services. In her study of diabetes in the elderly, Student 7 found a well organized primary health service centred around a rural village GP practice where a diabetic clinic was held once a week for two hours. Computerized, annual recall of patients operated and the practice nurse had completed the ENB 928 course on diabetic nursing. Health education and advice specific to each patient's needs was observed. In addition, district nurses held a daily clinic which patients with foot or leg ulcers could attend for dressings. The district nurses also visited patients in their own or residential homes for the administration of insulin to frail insulin-dependent diabetics unable to manage their own injections. Student 7 observed: 'The diabetic health care provision at the Health Centre is of a very high standard . . . . I observed close cooperation and good communication between all members of the primary health care team. They had an enthusiastic approach and were dedicated to meeting the needs of the diabetic patients in their care'. Even so, Student 7 found that there was a need for local chiropody services as, in a rural area, many of the elderly patients were not able to travel the necessary distance for this service. She also observed that a diabetic clinical nurse specialist could have offered periodic 'consultant' advice to professional staff in terms of updating their knowledge and skills, and in offering specific advice on the management of diabetes in patients who were experiencing particular difficulties.

## OUTCOMES

Students carrying out a local neighbourhood study as part of a learning process were not empowered to specify outcomes, goals or targets in relation to any particular allocation of resources. Nevertheless, it will have been observed in many of the extracts from the studies shown above just how aware the students were of the types of outcomes that they would specify in order to add 'life to years' for the groups selected for study within their neighbourhoods. Indeed, all the students concluded their studies with the recommendations that they would wish to make for improvements in their areas.

Student 4 who studied services for children with learning disabilities, found a particular difficulty for parents living in an area of great social deprivation. Services tend to be centralized because children with learning disabilities are a relatively small group which is widely dispersed geographically. For the parents in her neighbourhood this could mean major difficulties in terms of transport and communication. Through talking with families she found that perhaps the *greatest* need was for an information service which they could draw on in order to find out just what services they could expect either as a right, or subject to discretion. Too frequently, it appeared, that services could be available (for example, heating allowances, toys and appliances, and respite care) but parents were unsure of their eligibility and how to apply. Student 4 concluded that a more effective service could be provided if *all* health professionals learned more about the special needs of those with learning disabilities, and how to direct their carers to appropriate services. The desirable outcomes which she noted were therefore just as much concerned with the education and training of service providers as with characteristics in the recipients of their services.

## CONCLUSION

This chapter has been concerned with local health needs assessment by health visitors and undergraduate nurses in Nottingham. If one takes this local material and extrapolates from this the probability that similar exercises are going on around the UK, then the amount of health needs assessment by members of the nursing profession must be truly phenomenal. It appears that many of the requirements of contemporary government policy on health needs assessment are already being met by nurses. One must ask 'why does this material have such low visibility?' and 'to what extent are the findings applied either locally or elsewhere?' King's Fund NDU status funding for Strelley NDU has now expired. In future, the initiatives which have been developed there and which have been so influential in determining national policy, will be dependent on purchasers identifying a need for the services. Some may choose to assume that such public health work lies outside the 'proper' function of the nurse. Indeed, history suggests that it might not be long before such activities become defined as the province of an alternative form of worker (Davies 1988).

The undergraduate nursing students, in their turn, demonstrated through their Neighbourhood Studies an acute awareness of the relationship between economic, social, emotional and physical well being. They realized that many of the desirable outcomes were not achievable within the province of health services. On the other hand, they also saw that a great deal could be achieved through examples of best practice where team or inter-agency working was a reality and their recommendations reflected these insights.

# Conclusions and implications for nurses

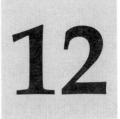

## INTRODUCTION

This has not been a 'how to do it' book but rather a book about conceptual frameworks and guiding ideas. Its aim has been to give nursing professionals some knowledge in sociology, epidemiology and economics in order to equip them with the tools to interpret and enter into the different debates surrounding health needs assessment. In particular, the book has aimed to give nurses an understanding of the complexity of the issues faced by government and purchasing authorities – such as District Health Authorities – in assessing health needs and developing priorities or targets for action. We hope that the book has also been of interest to other health care professionals.

We believe that there are three major challenges for nursing arising from our review of the issues surrounding the assessment of health needs. The first is that nurses working in provider units must be able to justify their work to local purchasing authorities such as District Health Authorities. They must be able to show that the work that they do is central to the ultimate aim of purchasing authorities of improving people's health. The second challenge is for nurses not only to provide evidence to purchasers that the services they provide do make a difference to people's health, but also to contribute to the work of purchasing authorities, providing an input into the assessment of need and the formulation of priorities for action. The third challenge is for nurses working on both sides of the purchaser/ provider split to participate in current theoretical debates. Nursing has an important contribution to make in questioning current ideas about needs assessment, and in ensuring that nursing values remain core values in health needs assessment. In the remainder of this chapter we discuss ways in which nurses have attempted to meet these challenges.

## SECTION I: DEMONSTRATING THE WORTH OF NURSING

### Introduction

We have seen in Chapters 4 and 10 that the purpose of the purchaser/provider split is that health authorities should determine their resource allocation on the basis of need. In the following section we look at the four main criteria used by Health Authorities in deciding which services to deliver in order to meet need. We look at the criteria of effectiveness; cost-effectiveness; equity; and consumer responsiveness. We argue that if the work of nurses in provider units is to be purchased by Health Authorities then they must respond to the challenge of meeting these criteria. Nurses must be able to show that the services they provide are both effective and cost-effective – that they do make a difference to people's health and that they provide value for money. Nurses have an important role to play too in ensuring that services are delivered equitably and in a way which is responsive to people's needs.

In this chapter we rely heavily on Shirley Goodwin's work (Goodwin 1992, 1994). Goodwin has done much excellent work in looking at the implications for comunity nurses of recent government policy.

### Effectiveness

One of the main challenges for nursing is to demonstrate to purchasers that their work is effective – that it succeeds in doing what it sets out to do. Despite the growth in the amount of information currently collected by Health Authorities as a result of the recent reforms, it is widely acknowledged that there is a lack of information about the outcomes, and therefore the effectiveness, of different medical and nursing interventions and different forms of service provision (for example community versus hospital care). Smith (1991c) has estimated that only about 15% of medical interventions are supported by solid scientific evidence. Similarly, few nursing interventions are supported by solid evidence (Barriball & MacKenzie 1993). Much of the information currently available about effectiveness, including nursing effectiveness, is the product not of 'hard' scientific evidence (for example clinical trials), but of so-called 'soft' evidence, that is, the experience of clinicians and nurses working in the area (Klein 1993).

Demonstrating the effectiveness of their work is a particularly hard task for nurses because many nursing interventions are non-clinical interventions, the effectiveness of which is much harder to measure than strictly clinical interventions which have hard and fast outcomes such as reducing mortality. Medical treatments with drugs are comparatively easy to measure. However, it is harder to measure the outcomes of much of the work carried out by nurses. Measuring the outcomes of health education, of providing psychological support to patients or carers, of providing social support to mothers, or of palliative care to the dying is not easy (Goodwin 1992). The effectiveness of many nursing interventions cannot be measured by such tangible indicators as mortality and morbidity rates. As we saw in Chapter 3, nursing often relies on less tangible (and often more holistic) indicators of positive health, such as indicators of psychological well-being, social integration and social support. We saw too in Chapter 3 that subjective health indicators are also vital for measuring nursing outcomes. For any kind of health care intervention there may be differences between the views of professionals and their clients about whether a particular intervention has resulted in a beneficial outcome. Thus, in assessing the outcome of much of the support work, counselling and education carried out by nurses the subjective views of clients about whether they feel they have benefited can be as valid a measure of the success of the intervention as any professionally-defined criterion of success. The difficulty of finding appropriate ways of measuring non-clinical outcomes is widely recognized and there is currently a great deal of work being carried out to devise relevant and appropriate measures of non-clinical outcomes, including nursing outcomes (see, for example, Holmes 1989, Long 1994, Brettle et al 1995).

. The difficulties involved in measuring nursing outcomes are not the only obstacle in demonstrating the effectiveness of nursing interventions. A further difficulty results from the fact that preventive nursing interventions frequently seek to achieve long-term, rather than short-term outcomes (Goodwin 1994). For example, as we saw in Chapter 5, the outcomes of much of the health promotion and prevention activities carried out by nurses in the child and school health services might only begin to be reflected in such outcome indicators as mortality rates half a century later.

Finally, it is often very difficult to demonstrate the effectiveness of nursing interventions because nursing outcomes are often crucially affected by factors other than nursing inputs. Nurses frequently work with the most deprived members of society and factors such as poverty and unemployment affect the outcomes of much of the work they do. As we saw in Chapter 11, it is not easy for health visitors working in a deprived area like Strelley to demonstrate that their work has brought about improved health outcomes for local people when poverty and deprivation are likely to counteract the beneficial effects of their work (Brummell & Perkins 1995).

Despite the difficulty of measuring the effectiveness of nursing interventions in terms of conventional 'hard' outcomes such as reductions in mortality and morbidity rates, or rates of service use, some work has been carried out, particularly in the USA, to demonstrate the effectiveness of nursing interventions in such terms. For example, in the hospital sector, work undertaken in the USA has suggested that the organization and quality of nursing care (nursing processes) can affect mortality rates (outcomes). A study undertaken by Aiken et al (1994) in the USA used the case–control method (described in Ch. 6) to compare mortality rates among Medicare patients at two groups of hospitals (Medicare is the American health insurance system providing cover for elderly persons). The first group of hospitals consisted of 39 'Magnet' hospitals which, prior to the study of Aiken et al, been singled out in a set of research studies as 'good' places to practise nursing (McClure et al 1983). The organization and quality of nursing care was considered to be of a high standard in these 39 hospitals. The second group (the 'controls') consisted of 195 other 'non-Magnet' hospitals which matched the 39 'case' hospitals in every other important respect (for example, they were of a similar size and had a similar ratio of doctors to patients) but had not been previously identified for their high quality nursing care. After adjusting for the difference in predicted mortality between the two sets of hospitals, the 39 'case' hospitals were found on average to have a 4.6% lower mortality rate among Medicare patients than the matched 'control' hospitals. Aiken et al (1994) concluded that 'The same factors that lead hospitals to be identified as effective from the standpoint of the organization of nursing care are associated with lower mortality among Medicare patients'.

In relation to community nursing, Ann Oakley (1993) has reviewed evidence of the effectiveness of the work of community nurses in terms of 'hard' indicators of outcome. Oakley has described a number of studies which have shown that social support offered by community nurses to mothers before and after birth has significantly improved both the physical and mental health of mothers, as well as the health of their children, and has so decreased their use of health services. One of the studies reviewed by Oakley was a randomized trial, conducted in America, of home visits to pregnant women most of whom were teenaged, unmarried and living in poverty. The study found that those who received a home visit from a health professional gave birth to heavier babies than those who received only the routine antenatal services. Among those who received a home visit there were fewer cases of child abuse and neglect, and fewer child accidents. The researchers thus concluded that home visiting can succeed in bringing about demonstrable improvements in physical and mental health, despite the effects of deprivation and the stressful environment in which many families live (Oakley 1993, Goodwin 1994).

## Cost-effectiveness

Cost-effectiveness (efficiency) is about getting value for money. Given that resources are scarce, it makes sense to purchasers to try to use their resources efficiently, and to ensure that costs do not rise to a level which cannot be afforded.

Clearly, an important cost to Health Authorities is the cost of nursing personnel. In attempting to get value for money, Health Authorities often rely on skill mix reviews which attempt to calculate how many nurses with particular skills and on particular pay grades are needed to carry out a given level of service. However, costs are only one-half of the cost-effectiveness equation. Cost-effectiveness involves relating costs to the outcomes of the services which are delivered – it involves relating inputs to outcomes. It is tempting to purchasers to try to simply reduce their costs by employing fewer highly-qualified nurses. The challenge to nurses is therefore to point to the link between the employment of more highly qualified (and therefore more expensive) nurses and better outcomes. This challenge has been taken up in a number of studies which have been reviewed by Hancock (1993). Perhaps the most important study reviewed by Hancock is a study undertaken by Bagust et al (1992) which found that 'good' nursing outcomes were dependent on the employment of highly-qualified nurses. This study concluded that reducing costs by employing fewer highly-qualified nurses would result in reduced effectiveness. Other studies reviewed by Hancock also suggested that nursing effectiveness is directly related to grade mix, so that a 'cost-minimization' approach to the employment of nursing personnel is likely to result in reduced effectiveness.

Given that resources are finite, purchasers must continually seek ways of achieving better, more effective, outcomes with the same level of resources. Hancock (1994) has described one of the ways in which existing nursing resources are being used more cost-effectively. She has drawn attention to the existence of number of 'hospital at home' schemes which offer intensive nursing in the home for people who might otherwise occupy expensive hospital beds. Such schemes have facilitated early discharge from hospital, unblocking beds and reducing waiting lists. Evaluation of a 'hospital at home' scheme which has been in operation in Peterborough since 1978 has shown that patients receiving care at home have been rehabilitated more quickly than patients who have received conventional postoperative care in hospital (Marks 1991). 'Hospital at home' schemes have thus provided clear evidence of both their effectiveness and cost-effectiveness. Moreover, such schemes have proved highly satisfactory to patients. Thus not only are such schemes cost-effective, they are also responsive to the wishes of clients.

## Equity

We have seen in Chapters 5 and 7 that equity is about distributing resources fairly. Horizontal equity means that those with equal needs should have equal access to services, and vertical equity means that those whose needs are greater should be targeted for extra resources in order to combat the 'inverse care law' (Goodwin 1994; see also Ch. 5).

Nurses have a major role to play in ensuring that services are delivered equitably. Much of the work that community nurses do is concerned with putting into practice the principle of vertical equity, that is, with attempting to improve the access to essential services of those deprived groups whose need is greatest. For example, the aim of the work undertaken at Strelley and described in Chapter 11 was to promote health gain among those deprived groups who do not always derive as much benefit from health care services as other groups. As we saw in Chapter 11, the focus of much of the work carried out in Strelley was on increasing the accessibility of services to a deprived local population. For example, much effort was devoted to increasing the uptake of child-health services and to reducing the disproportionate morbidity and mortality from accidents experienced by children in this locality. By working with local people to improve their access to essential services and to increase the material and information resources needed to reduce their risk of experiencing ill-health, the Strelley team were attempting to ensure that 'health gain' was distributed more equitably between deprived and more affluent localities within Nottingham Health Authority.

## Consumer-responsiveness

Consumer-responsiveness is about ensuring that services are not only cost-effective and equitable, but are also relevant, appropriate and sensitive to people's needs. It involves responding to what people themselves define as their needs, rather than to what professionals, purchasing authorities or governments may define as their needs.

The work undertaken in Strelley and described in Chapter 11 illustrates that there can be differences between the ways in which ordinary members of the community define their needs and the ways in which 'experts' define their needs. In Strelley, the health visiting team found that local people viewed with greatest concern such factors as the lack of nursery provision for the under-5s, a lack of safe play areas, a lack of welfare rights advice, and a lack of social support for young mothers experiencing the problems of isolation, loneliness and depression. Local people thus placed the greatest emphasis not on narrowly-defined health needs, but on their social and economic needs which arose from their poverty and deprivation. The Strelley public health workers recognized that if services were to be truly appropriate to people's needs then this involved addressing not only their health needs, but also those socio-economic factors which gave rise to poor physical and mental health. A fundamental aim of the work undertaken at Strelley was to address the effects of socio-economic factors such as poverty and low-income on health. For example, the Strelley team set up initiatives such as the 'safety equipment scheme' in which fireguards and safety gates could be purchased at a reduced cost because it was recognized that the price of safety equipment deterred those on low incomes from purchasing items which could reduce the risks of mortality and morbidity from accidents among children (Boyd et al 1993, Royal College of Nursing 1994). Thus, the recognition that poverty was a major barrier to the promotion of health gains was central to the provision of appropriate services to the people of Strelley. Many of the undergraduate nurses also observed in their Neighbourhood Studies the crucial link between poverty and its disabling effects on people's ability to participate meaningfully in society.

The Strelley team also believed that if services were to be appropriate and sensitive to people's needs, then this must involve a recognition that improving people's health involved more than exhorting them to adopt a healthier life-style. As we saw in Chapter 11, the Strelley team rejected the current emphasis by policy-makers on individual reponsibility for health because if fails to take account of those structural factors such as poverty, inadequate housing, and unemployment, which limit people's ability to make healthy choices.

Local people in Strelley did not experience their problems separately as 'health', 'social' and 'economic' problems, and therefore the most appropriate way of responding to their needs was to ensure collaboration between the various agencies involved in meeting need. The Strelley team did much work in facilitating an inter-agency approach, fostering collaboration between various professional groups and statutory and voluntary agencies in a way which addressed the totality of local people's health, social, and economic needs. The Strelley team were instrumental in setting up a number of multi-agency groups with representatives who could bring a range of perspectives to bear on the multiple problems experienced by local people.

The work of the Strelley team was based on the belief that clients are not simply passive recipients of services to meet their health and social needs. Being responsive to clients' needs means, above all, that clients can be empowered to become more active participants in their own care. The Strelley health workers contributed in a variety of ways to empowering local people. They supported local people in setting up and running various self help groups, such as the Women's Health and Leisure Group which was set up in response to the isolation and depression experienced by young mothers. Local people were also involved in many of the multi-agency groups, such as the Accident Prevention Group, and the Community Health Group.

Finally, the aim of being responsive to locally-defined needs raised a difficult dilemma for the Strelley health visitors. As we saw in Chapter 11, the stated aims of the Strelley NDU were both to respond to the needs expressed by local people themselves, and to work towards the achievement of national targets such as the *Health of the Nation* targets. (Brummell & Perkins 1995). These two sets of aims were not always compatible, and the Strelley team had to make difficult decisions about whether to pursue national targets or to respond to locally-defined needs. However, there did exist some common ground. One priority chosen for action in Strelley was child accident prevention. This was a target chosen in the *Health of the Nation* but it was also an issue which local people had highlighted as of central importance in their lives.

## SECTION 2: THE CONTRIBUTION OF NURSES TO PURCHASING AUTHORITIES

In this section we look at the ways in which nurses on both sides of the purchaser/provider divide can contribute to the assessment of need and the formulation of priorities for action at the level of the District Health Authority.

### Needs assessment

We saw in Chapters 1 and 4 that the government and the NHSME have issued many policy documents and directives concerned with enabling health authorities to assess needs. However, as we stressed in Chapter 11, there is little reference to the wealth of profile information concerning the health needs of local populations which has already been gathered by nurses (see also Goodwin 1992). District Health Authorities currently rely largely on assessments of need undertaken by Directors of Public Health. As we saw in Chapter 10, Directors of Public Health collect a great deal of data about health needs, such as morbidity and mortality data, data about health service activity, and demographic, social and economic data derived largely from the Census. However, the perspective of Directors of Public Health is essentially a 'top-down' perspective. Goodwin (1992) argues that nurses are often better placed than Directors of Public Health to take a 'bottom-up' perspective, gathering in-depth information about the nature of the problems experienced by ordinary people, thereby providing an additional dimension to the picture painted by the 'top-down' information contained in reports produced by Directors of Public Health. We, too, would argue that many of the community profiles and neighbourhood studies produced by nurses, including the studies produced by undergraduate nurses described in Chapter 11, could be used by Directors of Public Health to supplement their statistics with more detailed information how people experience their problems. For example, the neighbourhood study of local carers undertaken by a learner nurse and described in Chapter 11 (Student 8), which drew on the experiences of carers themselves, was able to highlight how carers experienced their health and social problems. This study was able to identify which services carers themselves viewed as best meeting their needs and where they felt there were gaps in service provision. Such 'bottom-up' information is vital to Directors of Public Health if they are to fulfil their aim of identifying unmet needs, and evaluating existing services to meet need.

Profiles of the health needs of the local population produced by nurses can also provide much valuable information about inequalities in health between different sections of the community. Such information is vital to the aim of promoting equity. Health Authorities need to know which groups suffer disproportionately from poor health in order to target resources on those in greater need. Much work has been done by nurses to document inequalities in health. For example, the public health work at Strelley began with the construction of a community profile of the area which documented the fact that Strelley was a disadvantaged area with high levels of poverty, unemployment, morbidity and mortality. Such information served as a justification for the Health Authority's decision to target health visiting resources towards Strelley (Jackson 1994). Similarly in Bristol, the department of public health medicine of the local Health Authority worked with local health visitors to find out who among the population had a high level of health risk, using indicators such as low income, unemployment, parental depression, poor housing and recent divorce, separation or bereavement (Shepherd 1992, Goodwin 1994).

Profiling exercises such as these provide vital information for decisions by purchasing authorities to target health resources, such as health visiting personnel, on deprived groups.

## Priority-setting

We have stressed throughout this book that in deciding on priorities, Health Authorities must take account not only of the effectiveness and cost-effectiveness of different interventions, they must also listen to the views of individuals and communities about which health outcomes they value, which services they view as beneficial, and which services they believe should have priority.

In attempting to take into account the priorities of consumers, District Health Authorities are often limited to relying on questionnaires of 'consumer satisfaction', or to organizing public meetings to which 'representatives' of the local community are invited. As we saw in Chapter 4, a danger in the kinds of public consultation exercises which the NHSME has recommended to District Health Authorities that they should undertake is that they may encourage those consumers most able to register their demands or needs to do so at the expense of those less able to articulate their needs. The NHSME has urged that District Health Authorities listen to 'local voices', (NHS Management Executive 1992; see also Ch. 4), but as Carroll (1994), a Director of Public Health employed by North Essex Health Authority points out, there are many 'silent voices' in the community – the housebound, the elderly and the poor – whose needs and wishes are not easily registered by the kinds of public consultation exercises advocated by the NHSME. Nurses, through their day-to-day contact with ordinary people, are uniquely placed to listen to the 'silent voices' in the community and to ensure that the consumer view is not restricted to the views of the most vociferous members of local communities.

Despite the difficulties which health authorities face in gaining a picture of the views and priorities of local people, real attempts to elicit the views of consumers have been made by some purchasing authorities (see Ong & Humphris 1994, Carroll 1994). One health authority (North-Essex) conducted a survey, in conjunction with Social Services, to gain an understanding of the important health issues that concerned members of one small rural community in Essex (Carroll 1994). As in Strelley, the concerns and priorities identified by local people in Essex did not neatly fit with the kinds of priorities or targets set out in the *Health of the Nation* or the *Patients' Charter*. Local people did not emphasize hospital-based services or the importance of reducing waiting lists. Their priorities could not be neatly categorized as 'coronary heart disease' or 'lung cancer'. Rather, ill-health was defined by local people far more widely than simply problems requiring hospital treatment, and respondents pointed to a whole spectrum of influences on their health. Responses to the interview survey carried out by North-Essex Health Authority included 'I am exhausted from caring for my elderly relative who can't get any real nursing support because the district nurses are run off their feet', and 'I am concerned about my teenagers smoking and taking drugs, and about my unemployed husband who is getting depressed because his employment prospects are going down month by month' (Carroll 1994). Thus, many of the priorities identified by local people went beyond the province of narrowly-defined health outcomes concerned only with adding 'years to life'. They required the health authority to take account of the structural causes of ill-health, and to acknowledge the importance of supportive interventions which do not necessarily add 'years to life'. They required too that the health authority should collaborate more closely with other agencies and departments, including Social Services, the police, education, and voluntary organizations.

The work undertaken by community nurses in Strelley illustrates the way in which nurses can bring to the attention of purchasing authorities the views and priorities of local people. In Strelley, as we saw above, local people's priorities did not fit easily with the priorities identified by governments. Consultation with local people in Strelley revealed that they did not employ a definition of their 'health needs' as the need for effective and cost-effective health care interventions. Like the local people in Essex, they employed a broader conception of health than the mere absence of disease. They did not give priority to narrow health-care interventions designed to reduce morbidity and mortality. Instead, they gave the highest priority to those interventions which enabled them to participate more fully in society. They valued supportive and empowering services which reduced the restrictions on their achieving better physical and social health.

Nurses involved in initiatives such as Strelley thus have an important role to play not only in responding to locally-defined needs but also in representing to purchasing authorities, including both Health and Local Authorities, the views of local people about which kinds of outcomes they value and which kinds of services they believe they have the greatest ability to benefit from.

The conclude, nurses have a vital role to play in providing a bottom-up perspective to complement the top-down approach of Directors of Public Health. They are well placed to provide information to purchasing authorities about how local people experience their problems, about what local people view as the most important influences on their health, and about which services ordinary people view as the most important. Such a bottom-up perspective is vital if needs assessment and the process of determining priorities is not to be dominated solely by concerns about adding years to life, and if purchasing authorities are to respond appropriately to the totality of people's health, social and economic needs.

## SECTION 3: CONCLUSIONS

In the following, final section we draw together material from throughout this book to summarize the ways in which we believe that nurses can challenge the bases on which governments and purchasing authorities assess health needs and determine priorities.

First, nursing has a role to play in challenging the dominant emphasis on curative rather than caring interventions. Despite widespread acknowledgement that caring interventions have a place in the delivery of effective and appropriate health care, government policy is nevertheless dominated by concerns about reducing mortality. As we saw above and in Chapter 4, this emphasis on 'cure' is reflected in the targets set in the government's *Health of the Nation* strategy which place an undue emphasis on adding 'years to life'. Nurses, whether working in purchaser or provider units, can play an important role in re-asserting the value of caring interventions. Interventions which directly reduce morbidity and mortality might have the most measurable and demonstrable outcomes, but governments and purchasing authorities should not be restricted by what is most measurable in deciding what kind of health benefits, curative or caring, should be pursued. We have seen above that it is very difficult to devise outcome measures by which to assess the effectiveness of much nursing work, but the difficulty of defining and measuring nursing outcomes is not a reflection of the worth of nursing's contribution. Nurses thus have a major role to play both in grappling with the very difficult task of demonstrating the effectiveness of what they do, but also in challenging the assumption that only those activities for which there exist hard and fast outcome measures and unequivocal evidence of their effectiveness are worth supporting.

Second, although inequalities in health, and in access to effective health care, have been a major concern to the international community for the past 25 years, they have been of less concern in recent British government policies. The current emphasis in British government policy is on the effectiveness and cost-effectiveness of interventions, with a lesser emphasis on questions of equity. In this country, policy-makers place great emphasis on the idea that services should be effective, and that resources should be used in ways which secure the best possible value for money. There is far less emphasis on the question of whether some groups in society are receiving their fair share of health care resources. The principle of equity was certainly a founding principle of the NHS, but it now takes second place. As we saw in Chapter 4, the goal of promoting equity played little part in the government's *Health of the Nation* strategy. The traditional concern of nursing has always been with equity. Nurses have always been concerned about the great differences in the health of the rich and the poor and about the poorer level of access and treatment afforded to deprived groups in society. It may be less cost-effective, less efficient, to target resources on the worst-off in society if they provide the least opportunity for achieving health gains, but efficiency should not be the most important criterion on which to base decisions about resource allocation. Nurses thus have an important role to play in continuing to bring to the attention of purchasing authorities evidence of inequalities in health and health care; in challenging those policies which are likely to benefit some groups in society more than others; and in working with deprived groups in society to improve their access to effective health care provision.

Third, nurses are all too aware of the limitations of the notion of individual responsibility for health. We saw above and in Chapters 4, 5 and 11 that it is a pervasive view among policy-makers that inequalities in health are the result of the unhealthy lifestyles adopted by some people. As we saw in Chapter 4, this explanation carried much weight in the government's *Health of the Nation* strategy which places great emphasis on the idea that individuals, through the adoption of a healthier lifestyle, can determine to a great extent their own health. Nurses, through their day-to-day contact with clients, are made constantly aware of the constraints many people face in making healthy 'choices'. Although nurses have an important role to play in continuing to provide health education and enabling people to adopt healthier lifestyles where they can, they cannot accept uncritically the notion that achieving health gains is solely a matter of educating people to make healthy choices. Nurses must challenge attempts on the part of governments and purchasing authorities to 'blame the victims' of poverty and inequality for their own poor health.

Finally, nurses believe they have an ethical 'duty of care'. They believe that as a society we should care for all those in need. Many economists, by constrast, are utilitarians. They believe there is an ethical imperative to implement only those health care services which are expected to lead to the best outcomes. QALYs are an expression of economists' utilitarian ethical principles.

We believe that nurses are right to feel distrustful of the QALY approach to setting priorities in health care in the sense that QALYs are interested only in the *outcomes* of services whereas nurses are interested in the plight of their patients, they are interested in the *process* of caring. QALYs may be one way of helping purchasers to decide on the most efficient use of resources, but they are not a means of deciding whether to respond to one person's health problems rather than another's. As Nord (1992) puts it, the difficulty with the QALY approach to health care policy-making is:

> its focus on quality of life in life-years rather than quality of life in people. In health care policy-making this is a somewhat strange and artificial perspective. The health services . . . . are concerned with providing care for living, breathing, feeling and thinking numbers, not with maximizing numbers of abstract time entities.

Nurses, like Nord (1992) and many others, believe that there is something wrong with a health service which pursues only outcomes to the extent of ignoring the actual suffering of real people (Doyal 1993, Chadwick 1994).

Nurses do not have a solution to the problem of rationing – to the problem that not all health care needs can be met – but they are right to emphasize that health care professionals have a moral duty of care.

Health care professionals cannot ignore the plight of their patients. Most nurses believe that poor health implies a moral right to at least some level of care, a right of access to whatever appropriate curative and caring interventions society has at its disposal, irrespective of whether such interventions are likely to prolong healthy life. Such beliefs cannot be lightly dismissed.

# References

Aiken L H, Smith H L and Lake E T ( 1994) Lower Medicare mortality amongst set of hospitals known for good nursing care. *Medical Care* 32: 771–787

Akehurst R and Ferguson B (1993) The Purchasing Authority, Chapter 9. In Drummond M F and Maynard A (eds) *Purchasing and Providing Cost-Effective Health Care.* Edinburgh: Churchill Livingstone

Akehurst R, Godfrey C, Hutton J and Robertson E (1991) *The Health of the Nation, An Economic Perspective on Target Setting,* Discussion Paper 92. Centre for Health Economics Health Economics Consortium, University of York

Bagust A, Slack R and Oakley J (1992) *Ward Nursing Quality and Grade Mix.* York Health Economics Consortium, University of York

Barclay P (1995) *Income and Wealth.* Rowntree Foundation Inquiry chaired by Sir Peter Barclay. York: Joseph Rowntree Foundation

Barker D J P and Osmond C (1992) Inequalities in Health in Britain: specific explanations in three Lancashire Towns. In Barker D J P (ed) *Fetal and Infant Origins of Adult Disease.* London: British Medical Journal

Barriball K L and MacKenzie A (1993) Measuring the impact of nursing interventions in the community: a selected review of the literature. *Journal of Advanced Nursing* 18: 401–407

Benzeval M, Blane D, Judge K, Marmot M, Power C, Whitehead M and Wilkinson R (1994) *Society and Health,* issue 1. London: King's Fund Institute and Centre for Health and Society

Benzeval M, Judge K and Whitehead M (eds) (1995) *Tackling Inequalities in Health: an Agenda for Action.* London: King's Fund

Billings J R and Cowley S (1995) Approaches to community needs assessment: a literature review. *Journal of Advanced Nursing* 22: 721–730

Black Sir D (1994) *A Doctor Looks at Health Economics.* Office of Health Economics Annual Lecture, London, OHE

Blackburn C (1991) *Poverty and Health: Working with Families.* Buckingham: OUP

Blackburn C (1992a) *Improving Health and Welfare Work with Families in Poverty: a Handbook.* Buckingham: OUP

Blackburn C (1992b) *Poverty Profiling.* London: Health Visitors Association

Blaxter, M (1985) Self-definition of health status and consulting rates in primary health care. *Quarterly Journal of Social Affairs* 1: 131–171

Bowling A (1992) *Measuring Health: a Review of Quality of Life Measurement Scales.* Buckingham: OUP

Boyd M (1993) Health visitors role out. *Nursing Standard* 47: 45–47

Boyd M, Brummell K, Billingham K and Perkins E R (1993) *The Public Health Post at Strelley: an Interim Report.* Nottingham Community Health NHS Trust. Nursing Development Units. London: King's Fund

Bradshaw J (1972a) The concept of social need. *New Society* 30 March 1972

Bradshaw J (1972b) A taxonomy of social need. In McLachlan G (ed) *Problems and Progress in Medical Care: Essays on current research,* 7th series. Buckingham: OUP

Bradshaw J (1994) The conceptualization and measurement of need: a social policy perspective, Chapter 3. In Popay J and Williams G (eds) *Researching the People's Health.* London: Routledge

Breeze E, Trevor G and Wilmot A (1991) *General Household Survey 1989,* OPCS Series GHS no 20. London: HMSO

Brettle A, Long A, Dixon P and Heaton J (eds) (1995) *An Introduction to Measuring Health Outcomes: an Annotated Bibliography.* Outcomes measurement bibliographies no 1, May 1995, Leeds, UK Clearing House on Health Outcomes, Nuffield Institute for Health, University of Leeds

British Medical Association (1987) *Deprivation and Ill-Health.* BMA Board of Science and Education Discussion Paper. London: BMA

Brown M and Madge N (1982) *Despite the Welfare State: a Report on the SSRC/DHSS Programme of Research in Transmitted Deprivation.* London: Heinemann Educational Books

Brummell K and Perkins E R (1995) *Public Health at Strelley: a Model in Action.* Nottingham Community Health NHS Trust, Nursing Development Units. London: King's Fund

Burghes (1980) *Living from Hand to Mouth: a Study of 65 Families Living on Suplementary Benefit.* London: Family Service Unit/Child Poverty Action Group

Burke P (1992) The ethics of screening, Chapter 4. In Hart C R and Burke P (eds) *Screening and Surveillance in General Practice.* Edinburgh: Churchill Livingstone

Burr M L and Elwood P C (1991) Research and development of health promotion services – screening. In Holland W W et al (eds) *Oxford Textbook of Public Health,* vol 3. Oxford: Oxford University Press

Campion M J, Cuzick J, McCance D J and Singer A (1986) Progressive potential of mild cervical atypia: prospective cytological, colposcopic and virological study. *Lancet* ii: 237–240

Carroll G (1994) Priority setting in purchasing health care, Chapter 13. In Smith R (ed) *Rationing in Action.* London: British Medical Journal Publishing Group

Carstairs V (1994) Health care needs, deprivation, and the resource allocation formula. In Gilman E, Munday S, Sommervaille L and Strachan R (eds) *Resource Allocation and Health Needs: from Research to Policy.* London: HMSO

Chadwick R (1994) Justice in priority setting, Chapter 8. In Smith R (ed) *Rationing in Action.* London: British Medical Journal Publishing Group

Challis L and Henwood M (1994) Equity in community care. *British Medical Journal* 308: 1496–1499

Chamberlain J M (1984) Which prescriptive screening programmes are worthwhile? *Journal of Epidemiology and Community Health* 38: 270–277

Clemen-Stone S, Eigsti D G and McGuire S L (1987) *Comprehensive Family and Community Health Nursing,* 2nd edn. New York: McGraw-Hill

Cochrane A L (1972) *Effectiveness and Efficiency: Random Reflections on Health Services.* London: Nuffield Provincial Hospitals Trust

Coulter A and Baldwin A (1987) Surveys of population coverage in cervical cancer screening in the Oxford Region. *Journal of the Royal College of General Practitioners* 37: 441–443

Council for the Education and Training of Health Visitors, 1965, Syllabus examination for health visitors in the United Kingdom. London: CETHV

Council for the Education and Training of Health Visitors, 1967, The Function of the Health Visitor. London: CETHV

Council for the Education and Training of Health Visitors, 1977, An investigation into the principles of health visiting. London: CETHV

Cowley S, Bergen A, Young K and Kavanagh A (1994) *The Changing Nature of Needs Assessment in Primary Health Care,* unpublished report on the initial stage of a project funded by the ENB, Department of Nursing Studies, King's College, London

Cuckle H S and Wald N J (1984) Principles of screening. In Wald N J (ed) *Antenatal and Neonatal Screening.* Buckingham: OUP

Culyer A J (1976) *Need and the National Health Service.* London: Martin Robertson

Culyer A J (1977) Need, values and health status measurement, Chapter 2. In Culyer A J and Wright K G (eds) *Economic Aspects of Health Services.* London: Martin Robertson

Culyer A J (1993) Chapter 17. In Van Doorslaer et al (eds) *Equity in the Finance and Delivery of Health Care: an International Perspective.* Oxford: Oxford Medical Publications

Dahlgren G and Whitehead M (1992) *Policies and Strategies to Promote Equity in Health.* Copenhagen: WHO Regional Office for Europe

Dale A and Marsh C (eds) (1993) *The 1991 Census User's Guide.* London: HMSO

Davies C (1988) The health visitor as mother's friend: a woman's place in public health, 1900–1914. *Social History of Medicine* 1: 39–59

Delamothe T (1991) Social class inequalities in health. *British Medical Journal* 303: 1046–1050

Department of Health (1989a) *Caring for People: Community Care in the Next Decade and Beyond.* London: HMSO

Department of Health (1989b) *Working for Patients*. London: HMSO

Department of Health (1990) *The NHS and Community Care Act* London: HMSO

Department of Health (1991a) *The Health of the Nation: a Consultative Document for Health in England*, Cm1523. London: HMSO

Department of Health (1991b) *Research for Health: a Research and Development Strategy for the NHS*. London: Department of Health

Department of Health (1992) *The Health of the Nation: a Strategy for Health in England*, Cm1986. London: HMSO

Department of Health (1993a) *Report of the Taskforce on the Strategy for Research in Nursing, Midwifery and Health Visiting*. London: Department of Health

Department of Health (1993b) *The Health of the Nation: Working Together for Better Health*. London: Department of Health

Department of Health (1994a) *Report on the State of the Public Health: the Annual Report of the Chief Medical Officer of the Department of Health for the Year 1993*. London: HMSO

Department of Health (1994b) *The challenges for Nursing and Midwifery in the 21st Century. The Heathrow Debate, 1993*. London: Department of Health

Department of Health (1995a) *Health of the Young Nation: Your Contribution Counts*. Report of two Nursing Conferences – January and February 1995. London: Department of Health

Department of Health (1995b) *On the State of the Public Health 1994*. London: HMSO

Department of Public Health (1995c) *Variations in Health: What Can the Department of Health and the NHS do?* A report of the Variations Sub-group of the Chief Medical Officer's Health of the Nation Working Group. London: Department of Health

Doll Sir R (1992) Address to 'The Burden of Cancer'. Nottingham: Nottingham School of Public Health

Donabedian A (1980) *Explorations in Quality Assessment and Monitoring*, vol 1: *the Definition of Quality and Approaches to its Assessment*. Ann Arbor, MI: Health Administration Press

Donaldson C (1994) Economics of priority setting: let's ration rationally! Chapter 7. In Smith R (ed) *Rationing in Action*. London: British Medical Journal Publishing Group

Downie R S and Calman K C (1994) *Healthy Respect: Ethics in Health Care*. Oxford: Oxford Medical Publications

Downie J and Elstein A (eds) (1988) *Professional judgement: a Reader in Clinical Decision making*, pp 1–41. Cambridge: Cambridge University Press

Downie R S, Fyfe C and Tannahill A (1994) *Health Promotion: Models and Values*. Buckingham: OUP

Doyal L (1993) The role of the public in health care rationing *Critical Public Health* 4: 49–54

Doyal L and Gough I (1992) *A Theory of Human Need*. Hampshire and London: MacMillan Press Ltd

Drummond M F (1978) Evaluation and the National Health Service, Chapter 5. In Culyer A J and Wright K G (eds) *Economic Aspects of Health Services*. London: Martin Robertson

Drummond M F (1993) The contribution of health economics to cost-effective health care delivery, Chapter 2. In Drummond M F and Maynard A (eds) *Purchasing and Providing Cost-Effective Health Care*. Edinburgh: Churchill Livingstone

Drummond M F, Stodart G I and Torrance G W (1994) *Methods for the Economic Evaluation of Health Care Programmes*. Oxford: Oxford Medical Publications

Farmer R and Miller D (1991) *Lecture Notes on Epidemiology and Public Health Medicine*. Oxford: Blackwell Scientific Publications

Finnegan L and Ervin N (1989) An epidemiological approach to community assessment. *Public Health Nursing* 6: 3, 147–151

Fitzpatrick R (1995) Health needs assessment, chronic illness and the social sciences, Chapter 10. In *Researching the People's Health*. Poppay J and Williams G (eds) London: Routledge

Fox H (1987) Cervical smears: new terminology and new demands. *British Medical Journal* 294: 1307–1308

Frankenberg R (1969) *Communities in Britain: Social Life in Town and Country.* Harmondsworth: Pelican/Pelican

Frater A and Sheldon T A (1993) The outcomes movement in the USA and the UK, Chapter 4. In Drummond M F and Maynard A (eds) *Purchasing and Providing Cost-Effective Health Care.* Edinburgh: Churchill Livingstone

French B (1995) The role of outcomes in the measurement of nursing. *Nurse Researcher* 2: 4, 5–13

Friedman G D (1980) *Primer of Epidemiology,* 2nd edn. New York: McGraw-Hill

Friedman G D (1985) Entry under 'Epidemiology'. In Kuper A and Kuper J (eds) *The Social Science Encyclopedia.* London: Routledge and Kegan Paul

Fullard E, Fowler G and Gray M (1987) Promoting prevention in primary care: controlled trial of low technology, low cost approach. *British Medical Journal* 294: 1080–1082

Gibson T C (1966) Community health services in the management of congestive heart failure. *Journal of Chronic Disease* 19: 133

Gilbert J (1993) Close encounters. *Nursing Times* 89: 50–51

Gilman E, Sommervaille L and Griffiths R K (1994) Deprivation and resource allocation in the West Midlands Regional Health Authority, p. 19. In Gilman E, Munday S, Sommervaille L and Strachan R (eds) *Resource Allocation and Health Needs: From Research to Policy.* London: HMSO

Goldacre M J and Vessey M P (1987) Health and sickness in the community. In Weatherall D J et al (eds), *Oxford Textbook of Medicine,* 2nd edn. Oxford: OUP

Goodwin S (1991) Breaking the links between social deprivation and poor child health. *Health Visitor* 64: 376–379

Goodwin S (1992) Crossing the purchaser/provider divide. *Health Visitor* 65: 78–80, reproduced in *A Power of Good: Health Visiting in the 1990s,* Health Visitors' Association, 1994

Goodwin S (1994) Purchasing effective care for parents and young children. *Health Visitor* 67: 127–129, reproduced in *A Power of Good: Health Visiting in the 1990s,* Health Visitors' Association, 1994

Gough I (1992) What are human needs? Chapter 1. In Percy-Smith J and Sanderson I (eds) *Understanding Local Needs.* London: Institute of Public Policy Research, Premier Printers

Graham H (1984) *Women, Health and the Family.* Hemel Hempstead: Harvester Wheatsheaf

Greenfield S, Stillwell B and Drury M (1987) Practice nurses: social and occupational characteristics. *Journal of the Royal College of General Practitioners* 37: 341–345

Gregory J, Foster K, Tyler H and Wiseman M (1990) *The Dietary and Nutritional Survey of British Adults: a Survey Carried out by the Social Survey Division of OPCS with Dietary and Nutritional Evaluations by the Ministry of Agriculture, Fisheries and Food and the Department of Health.* London: HMSO

Grimes D S (1988) Value of a negative cervical smear. *British Medical Journal* 296: 1363

Hancock C (1993) Nurses work-cost effectively. *Nursing Standard* 7: no 26, 24–26

Hancock C (1994) Getting a quart out of a pint pot, Chapter 2. In Smith R (ed) *Rationing in Action.* London: British Medical Journal Publishing Group

Harris J (1985) *The Value of Life.* London: Routledge and Kegan Paul

Hart J T (1971) The Inverse Care Law. *Lancet* i: 405–412, reprinted in Cox C and Mead A (eds) (1975) *A Sociology of Medical Practice.* London: Collier McMillan

Hart J T (1987) *Hypertension,* 2nd edn. Edinburgh: Churchill Livingstone

Hart C R (1992) Theory and its application, Chapter 2. In Hart C R and Burke P (eds) *Screening and Surveillance in General Practice.* Edinburgh: Churchill Livingstone

Hawtin M, Hughes G and Percy-Smith J (1994) *Community Profiling: Auditing Social Needs.* Buckingham: OUP

Health Visitors Association School Nurse Sub-committee (1992) *Profiling School Health.* London: Health Visitors' Association

Helliwell B and Drummond M F (1988) The costs and benefits of preventing influenza in Ontario's elderly. *Canadian Journal of Public Health* 79: May/June 1988; 175–180

Holland W W (1983) *Evaluation and Health Care*. Oxford: Oxford University Press

Holland W W and Gilderdale S (eds) (1977) *Epidemiology and Health*. London: Kimpton

Holland W W and Karhausen L (eds) (1978) *Health Care and Epidemiology*. London: Kimpton

Holland W W and Stewart S (1990) *Screening in Health Care: Benefit or Bane*? London: The Nuffield Provincial Hospitals Trust

Holmes C A (1989) Health care and the quality of life: a review. *Journal of Advanced Nursing* 14: 833–839

Hudson T W, Reinhart M A, Rose S D and Stewart G K (1988) *Clinical Preventive Medicine*. Boston: Little, Brown and Co

Illsley (1987) Occupational class, selection and inequalities in health. *Quarterly Journal of Social Affairs* 3: 213–223

Irving D (1985) How to identify the needy. *Health and Social Service Journal* 95: 4929, January 3, 18–19

Jackson C (1994) Working together for health. *Health Visitor* 67: 28–29, reproduced in *A Power of Good: Health Visiting in the 1990s*, Health Visitors' Association, 1994

Jacobson B, Smith A and Whitehead M (eds) (1991) *The Nation's Health: A Strategy for the 1990s*. London: King Edward's Hospital Fund for London

Jarman B (1983) Identification of underprivileged areas. *British Medical Journal* 286: 1705–1709

Jarman B (1984) Underprivileged areas: validation and distribution of scores. *British Medical Journal* 289: 1587–1592

Jarman B and Bajekal M (1994) Resource allocation to fundholding practices, p. 33. In Gilman E, Munday S, Sommervaille L and Strachan R (eds) *Resource Allocation and Health Needs: from Research to Policy*, London: HMSO

Jenkins R (1990) Towards a system of outcome indicators for mental health care. *Journal of Psychiatry* 157: 500–514

Joseph Sir K (1972) Speech given at a conference organized by the Pre-School Playgroups Association reprinted in Butterworth E and Holman R (eds) *Social Welfare in Modern Britain*. Glasgow: Fontana/Collins

Judge K and Mays N (1994) Allocating resources for health and social care in England. *British Medical Journal* 308: 1363–1366

Kind P, Rosser R and Williams A (1982) Valuation of the quality of life: some psychometric evidence. In Jones-Lee M W (ed) *The Value of Life and Safety*. Amsterdam: North-Holland

Kirk E P (1993) The Oregon Experience, Chapter 2. In Tunbridge M (ed) *Rationing of Health Care in Medicine*. London: Royal College of Physicians

Klarman H E, Francis J O'S and Rosenthal G D (1968) Cost effectiveness analysis applied to the treatment of chronic renal failure. *Medical Care* 6: 48–54

Klein R (1988) Acceptable Inequalities? In Green D (ed) *Essays on the Pursuit of Equality in Health Care*. London: Institute for Economic Affairs Health Unit

Klein R (1991) Making Sense of Inequalities: a response to Peter Townsend. *International Journal of Health Services* 21: 175–181

Klein R (1993) Rationality and rationing: diffused or concentrated decision making? Chapter 8. In Tunbridge M (ed) *Rationing of Health Care in Medicine*. London: Royal College of Physicians

Kunst A E and Mackenbach J P (1994) *Measuring Socio-economic Inequalities in Health*. Copenhagen: WHO Regional Office for Europe

*Lancet* (1985) Cancer of the cervix – death by incompetence. Editorial, *Lancet* ii: 363–364

Lang T, Andres C, Bedale C, Hannon E and Hulme J (1984) *Jam Tomorrow*? Food Policy Unit, Manchester Polytechnic

Le Grand J (1987) Equity, Health, and Health Care. *Social Justice Research* 1: no 3

Leventhal B, Moy C and Griffin J (1993) *Market Research Society Census Interest Group*, An introductory guide to the 1991 Census. Henley on Thames: NTC Publications Ltd

Lightfoot J (1995) Identifying needs and setting priorities: issues of theory, policy and practice. *Health and Social Care* 3: 105–114

Long A (1994) Assessing health and social outcomes, Chapter 9. In Popay J and Williams G (eds) *Researching the People's Health*. London: Routledge

McAvoy B R and Raza R (1988) Contraceptive service and cervical cytology. *Health Trends* 20: 14–17

McClure M, Poulin M, Solvie M and Wandelt M (1983) *Magnet Hospitals: Attraction and Retention of Professional Nurses*, Task Force on Nursing Practice in Hospitals. Kansas City: American Nurses' Association

McKeown T (1979) *The Role of Medicine: Dream, Mirage, or Nemisis?* Oxford: Blackwell

McKeown T and Lowe C R (1966) *An Introduction to Social Medicine*. Philadelphia: Davies

MacMahon B and Pugh T F (1970) *Epidemiology – Principles and methods*. Boston: Little, Brown

Mant D and Fowler G (1990) Mass screening: theory and ethics. *British Medical Journal* 300: 916–918

Marks L (1991) *Home and Hospital Care: Re-drawing the Boundaries*. London: King's Fund

Marsh G N, Channing D M (1988) Narrowing the gap between a deprived and an endowed community. *British Medical Journal* 296: 173–176

Mascie-Taylor C G N (1990) The biology of social class. In Mascie-Taylor C G N (ed) *Biosocial Aspects of Social Class*. Oxford: Oxford University Press

Mausner J S and Bahn A K (1974) *Epidemiology: an Introductory Text*. Philadelphia: W B Saunders Co

Maynard A (1993) The economics of rationing health care, Chapter 1. In Tunbridge M (ed) *Rationing of Health Care in Medicine*. London: Royal College of Physicians of London

Mooney G (1992) *Economics, Medicine and Health Care*, 2nd edn. Hemel Hempstead: Harvester Wheatsheaf

Mooney G (1994) *Key Issues in Health Economics*. Hemel Hempstead: Harvester Wheatsheaf

Morris R and Carstairs V (1991) Which deprivation? – a comparison of selected deprivation indexes. *Journal of Public Health Medicine* 13: 318–326

Morris J K, Cook D G and Shaper A G (1994) Loss of employment and mortality. *British Medical Journal* 308: 1135–1139

Moser K A, Fox A J and Jones D R (1986) Unemployment and mortality in the OPCS Longitudinal Study. In Wilkinson R G (ed) *Class and Health: Research and Longitudinal Data*. London: Tavistock Publications Ltd

National Association of Health Authorities and Trusts (1995) *Making it Happen*, briefing, no. 81, May

NHS Executive (1994) *Building a Stronger Team: the Nursing Contribution to Purchasing*. A report on the impact of nursing skills and experience on the purchasing process. Leeds: NHSE

NHS Management Executive (1991) *Assessing Health Care Needs*. A DHA project discussion paper, May 1991. London: NHSME

NHS Management Executive (1992) *Local voices. The Views of Local People in Purchasing for Health*. London: NHMSE

NHS Management Executive (1993a) *A Vision for the Future: the Nursing, Midwifery and Health Visiting Contribution to Health and Health Care*. Leeds: Department of Health

NHS Management Executive (1993b) *New World, New Opportunities: Nursing in Primary Health Care*. Leeds: Department of Health

NHS Management Executive (1993c) *The Health of the Nation. Local Target Setting: a Discussion Paper*. Leeds: Department of Health

NHS Management Executive (1993d) *The Health of the Nation. Targeting practice: the Contribution of Nurses, Midwives and Health Visitors*. London: Department of Health

Nord E (1992) An alternative to QALYs: the saved young life equivalent (SAVE). *British Medical Journal* 305: 875–877

Nottingham Community Health NHS Trust (1993) *Strelley Nurse Development Unit, Health Visiting, Annual Report 1992–1993*. London: Nursing Development Units, King's Fund

Nottingham Community Health NHS Trust (1994) *Changing Needs: Changing Minds Changing Practice. Strelley Nurse Development Unit, Health Visiting, Annual Report 1994*. London: Nursing Development Units, King's Fund

Nottingham Health Authority (1990) *Annual Report on the Health of the People of Nottingham*. Nottingham Health Authority

Nottingham Health Authority (1991) *Annual Report on the Health of the People of Nottingham*. Nottingham Health Authority

Nottingham Health Authority (1992) *Annual Report on the Health of the People of Nottingham*. Nottingham Health Authority

Nottingham Health Authority (1993) *Annual Report on the Health of the People of Nottingham*. Nottingham Health Authority

Nottingham Health Authority (1995) *Annual Report on the Health of the People of Nottingham*. Nottingham Health Authority

Nottingham City Council (1994) *Poverty in Nottingham*, Policy Unit, Nottingham City Council

Nottinghamshire County Council Planning and Economic Development (1993) *Ward Unemployment September 1993*, Department of Planning and Economic Development, Trent Bridge House, Nottingham, NG2 6BJ

Nottinghamshire County Council, (1994) *Social Need in Nottinghamshire. County Disadvantaged Area Study 1994, Part 1*. Nottinghamshire County Council Planning and Economic Development

Nottinghamshire Structure Plan (1983) *Disadvantage in Nottinghamshire County Deprived Area Study 1983, Part I*

Oakley A (1993) *Social Support and Maternity and Child Health Care: a Guide to Good Quality Practice for NHS Purchasers*. Salford: Public health research and resources centre

Office of Health Economics (1995) Compendium of Health Statistics, 9th edn. London: OHE

Ong B N and Humphris G (1994) Prioritizing needs with communities, Chapter 4. In Popay J and Williams G (eds) *Researching the People's Health*. London: Routledge

Padden S C R (ed) (1993) A guide to health service statistics. Cheadle: Information for Management Health Care

Paton C R (1992) The economics of screening, Chapter 3. In Hart C R and Burke P (eds) *Screening and Surveillance in General Practice*. Edinburgh: Churchill Livingstone

Percy-Smith J and Sanderson I (1992) *Understanding Local Needs*. London: Institute for Public Policy Research (IPPR), Premier Printers

Phillimore P, Beattie A and Townsend P (1994) Widening inequality of health in Northern England, 1981–91. *British Medical Journal* 308: 1125–1128

Pickin C and St Leger S (1994) *Assessing Health Needs Using the Life Cycle Framework*. Buckingham: OUP

Pitkeathley J (1989) *It's my Duty isn't it? The Plight of Carers in our Society*. London: Souvenir Press

Pollock A (1992) Local voices. *British Medical Journal* 305: 535–536

Power C (1994) Health and social inequality in Europe. *British Medical Journal* 308: 1153–1156

Power C, Manor O and Fax J (1991) *Health and Class: the Early Years*. London: Chapman and Hall

*Public Health in England: The Report of the Committee of Inquiry into the Future Development of the Public Health Function* (1988), Cm 289. London: HMSO

Radical Statistics Health Group (1991) Missing: a strategy for the health of the nation. In *The Health of the Nation: the BMJ View*. London: British Medical Journal Publishing Group

Raftery J and Stevens A (1994) Information for purchasing, Chapter 8. In Ham C and Heginbotham C (eds) *Information Management in Health Services*. Buckingham: OUP

Raphael D D (1981) *Moral Philosophy*. Buckingham: OUP

Reading R, Colver A, Openshaw S and Jarvis S (1994) Do interventions that improve immunisation uptake also reduce social inequalities in uptake? *British Medical Journal* 308: 1142–1144

Richardson (1994) Health needs assessment and resource allocation policy: which comes first? In Gilman E, Munday S, Sommervaille L and Strachan R (eds) *Resource Allocation and Health Needs: from Research to Policy*. London: HMSO

Ridsdale L (1992) Screening for carcinoma of the cervix, Chapter 24. In Hart C and Burke P (eds) *Screening and Surveillance in General Practice*. Edinburgh: Churchill Livingstone

Roberts C J, Charney M C, Farrow S C (1985) How much can the NHS afford to spend to save a life or avoid a severe disability? *Lancet i*: 89–91

Robertson J H, Woodend B E, Crozier E H, Hutchinson J (1988) Risk of cervical cancer associated with mild dyskaryosis. *British Medical Journal* 297: 18–21

Robinson J J A, Sowden A J and Tattersall R B (1995) The management of diabetes in adolescents and young adults: a preliminary case study. *Journal of Clinical Nursing* 4: 249–265

Robson J and Spiegal N (1992) Health teams: the preventive interface, Chapter 7. In Hart C R and Burke P (eds) *Screening and Surveillance in General Practice*. Edinburgh: Churchill Livingstone

Rose G and Barker D J P (1986) *Epidemiology for the Uninitiated*. London: British Medical Journal Publishing Group

Rosser R M and Kind P (1978) A scale of valuations of states of illness – is there a social consensus? *International Journal of Epidemiology* 7: 347–358

Rosser R M and Watts V C (1972) The measurement of hospital output. *International Journal of Epidemiology* 1: 361–368

Rosser R M, Cottee M, Rabin R and Selai C (1992) Index of health-related quality of life, pp 81–89. In Hopkins A (ed) *Measures of the Quality of Life*. London: Royal College of Physicians

Royal College of Nursing (1991a) *The Health of the Nation: Outline of RCN Response*, draft response to the Health of the Nation Green Paper. London: RCN

Royal College of Nursing (1991b) *Health of the Nation: a Response from the Royal College of Nursing* HSPC/91/66. London: RCN

Royal College of Nursing (1994) *Public Health: Nursing rises to the challenge*. London: RCN

Ryan N (1983) The epidemiological method of building causal inference. *Advances in Nursing Science* 5: 2; 73–81

Sackett D L and Holland W W (1975) Controversy in the detection of disease. *Lancet ii*: 357–359

Seedhouse D (1993) *Ethics: the Heart of Health Care*. Chichester: John Wiley

Seedhouse D (1994) *Health: the Foundations for Achievement*. Chichester: John Wiley

Sen A (1985) *Commomodities and Capabilities*. Amsterdam: Elsevier

Sen A (1992) *On Ethics and Economics*. Oxford: Blackwell

Shepherd M (1992) Comparing needs with resource allocation. *Health Visitor* 65: 303–306

Skrabanek P (1988) The physician's responsibility to the patient. *Lancet i*: 1155–1156

Smith R (1991a) First steps towards a strategy for health. In *The Health of the Nation: the BMJ View*. London: British Medical Journal Publishing Group

Smith R (1991b) Rationing: the search for sunlight. *British Medical Journal* 303: 1561–1562

Smith R (1991c) Where is the wisdom . . . . ? *British Medical Journal* 303: 798–799

Smyth T (1992) *Caring for Older People*. London: MacMillan Press

Snow J (1855) *On the Mode of Communication of Cholera*, 2nd ed. London: Churchill. Reproduced in *Snow on Cholera* (1936) Commonwealth Fund, New York. Reprinted by Hafner Publishing Company, New York, 1936

Spriggs A and Boddington M M (1976) Protection by cervical smears. *Lancet i*: 143

Standing P and Mercer S (1984) Quinquennial cervical smears: every woman's right and every practitioner's responsibility. *British Medical Journal* 289: 883–886

Standing Nursing and Midwifery Advisory Committee (1995), *Making it Happen: Public Health – the Contribution of Nurses, Midwives and Health Visitors.* London: Department of Health

Stevens A and Gabbay J (1991) Needs assessment needs assessment . . . . *Health Trends* 23: no 1, 20–23

Stirland H and Raftery J (1992) Wandsworth Health Authority Mental Health Needs Profile. In Griffiths S, Wylie I and Jenkins R (eds) *Creating a Common Profile for Mental Health.* Department of Health, London: HMSO

Stoate H (1989) Can health screening damage your health? *Journal of the Royal College of General Practitioners* 39: 193–195

Teeling Smith G (1975) The economics of screening, Chapter 3. In Hart C R (ed) *Screening in General Practice.* Edinburgh: Churchill Livingstone

Townsend P and Davidson N (eds) (1992) *Inequalities in Health: The Black Report and The Health Divide.* London: Penguin

Townsend P, Philimore P and Beattie A (1988) *Health and Deprivation: Inequality and the North.* London: Croom Helm

Twinn S, Dauncey J and Carnell J (1990) *The process of Health Profiling.* London: Health Visitors' Association

UKCC (1986) *Project 2000: a New Preparation for Practice.* London: UKCC

UKCC 1994 *The Future of Professional Practice – the Council's Standards for Education and Practice following Registration.* London: UKCC

Valanis B (1986) *Epidemiology in Nursing and Health Care.* Norwalk: Appleton-Century-Crofts

Walker D (1992) Are QALYs going to be useful to me as a purchaser of health services? pp 53–59. In Hopkins A (ed) *Measures of the Quality of Life.* London: Royal College of Physicians

Welsh Office (1995) *Towards Evidence Based Practice: a Clinical Effectiveness Initiative for Wales.* Cardiff: Welsh Office

Westcott G, Svensson P G and Zollner H F K (eds) (1985) *Health Policy Implications of Unemployment.* Copenhagen: WHO Regional Office for Europe

Whitehead M (1994) Who cares about equity in the NHS? *British Medical Journal* 308: 1284–1287

Whitehead M (1995) Tackling inequalities: a review of policy initiatives, Chapter 3. In Benzeval M, Judge K and Whitehead M (eds) *Tackling Inequalities in Health: an Agenda for Action.* London: King's Fund

Wilkinson R G (1992) Income distribution and life-expectancy. *British Medical Journal* 308: 1135–1139

Wilkinson R G (1994) Health, redistribution and growth. In Miliband D and Glyn A (eds) *Paying for Inequality: the Economic Costs of Social Injustice.* London: Rivers Oram Press

Williams A (1985a) Economics of coronary artery bypass grafting. *British Medical Journal* 291: 327–329

Williams A (1985b) The value of QALYs. *Health and Social Services Journal* 94: 4957 (suppl.); 3–4

Williams A (1993a) Economics, society and health care ethics, pp 829–842. In Gillon R and Lloyd A *Principles of Health Care Ethics.* Chichester: Wiley

Williams A (1993b) Equity in health care: the role of ideology, Chapter 16. In van Doorslaer E et al (eds) *Equity in the Finance and Delivery of Health Care: an International Perspective.* Oxford: Oxford Medical Publications

Williams A and Kind P (1992) The present state of play about QALYs, pp 21–34. In Hopkins A (ed) *Measures of the Quality of Life.* London: Royal College of Physicians

Wilson J and Junger G (1968) *Principles and Practice of Screening for Disease.* Public Health Papers WHO no 34. Geneva: WHO

Wilson S and Walker G M (1993) Unemployment and health: a review. *Public Health* 107: 153–162

Windmall V (1992) *Ageing Today: an Approach to Caring for the Elderly.* Bath: Bath Press

Winkelstein W Jr (1972) Epidemiological considerations underlying the allocation of health and disease care resources *International Journal of Epidemiology.* 1: 69–74

Woodroffe C, Glickman M, Barker M and Power C (1993) *Children, Teenagers and Health: the Key Data.* Buckingham: OUP

World Health Organization (WHO) (1994) *Basic Documents,* 40th edn. Geneva: World Health Organization, p 1–18

# Index